Making Sense

Making Sense of the ICD-11

For Mental Health Professionals

Edited by
Peter Tyrer
Emeritus Professor of Community Psychiatry, Imperial College London

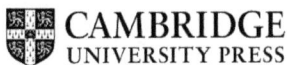

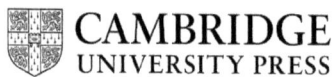

Shaftesbury Road, Cambridge CB2 8EA, United Kingdom

One Liberty Plaza, 20th Floor, New York, NY 10006, USA

477 Williamstown Road, Port Melbourne, VIC 3207, Australia

314–321, 3rd Floor, Plot 3, Splendor Forum, Jasola District Centre, New Delhi – 110025, India

103 Penang Road, #05–06/07, Visioncrest Commercial, Singapore 238467

Cambridge University Press is part of Cambridge University Press & Assessment, a department of the University of Cambridge.

We share the University's mission to contribute to society through the pursuit of education, learning and research at the highest international levels of excellence.

www.cambridge.org
Information on this title: www.cambridge.org/9781009182249

DOI: 10.1017/9781009182232

© Peter Tyrer 2023

This publication is in copyright. Subject to statutory exception and to the provisions of relevant collective licensing agreements, no reproduction of any part may take place without the written permission of Cambridge University Press & Assessment.

First published 2023

A catalogue record for this publication is available from the British Library.

A Cataloging-in-Publication data record for this book is available from the Library of Congress.

ISBN 978-1-009-18224-9 Paperback

Cambridge University Press & Assessment has no responsibility for the persistence or accuracy of URLs for external or third-party internet websites referred to in this publication and does not guarantee that any content on such websites is, or will remain, accurate or appropriate.

....

Every effort has been made in preparing this book to provide accurate and up-to-date information that is in accord with accepted standards and practice at the time of publication. Although case histories are drawn from actual cases, every effort has been made to disguise the identities of the individuals involved. Nevertheless, the authors, editors, and publishers can make no warranties that the information contained herein is totally free from error, not least because clinical standards are constantly changing through research and regulation. The authors, editors, and publishers therefore disclaim all liability for direct or consequential damages resulting from the use of material contained in this book. Readers are strongly advised to pay careful attention to information provided by the manufacturer of any drugs or equipment that they plan to use.

Contents

List of Contributors vi

Introduction: A Guide to This Book 1
Peter Tyrer

1 **Development and Innovation in the ICD-11 Chapter on Mental, Behavioural and Neurodevelopmental Disorders** 5
Geoffrey M. Reed

2 **ICD-11 + DSM-5 = A Diagnostic Babel** 17
Allen Frances

3 **Schizophrenia or Other Primary Psychotic Disorders** 25
Wolfgang Gaebel & Eva Salveridou-Hof

4 **Mood Disorders** 39
Gin S. Malhi & Erica Bell

5 **Disorders Specifically Associated with Stress** 59
Chris R. Brewin & Andreas Maercker

6 **Disorders Due to Substance Use** 70
John B. Saunders

7 **Child and Adolescent Psychiatric Disorders** 86
M. Elena Garralda

8 **Anxiety and Fear-Related Disorders and Obsessive-Compulsive and Related Disorders** 97
Dan J. Stein, Cary S. Kogan, & Christine Lochner

9 **Personality Disorders** 110
Roger Mulder

10 **Disorders of Intellectual Development** 122
Sally-Ann Cooper & Cary S. Kogan

11 **Eating Disorders** 135
Ulrike Schmidt

12 **Mental Health Classifications in Primary Care** 137
Christopher Dowrick

Index 145

Contributors

Erica Bell
Academic Department of Psychiatry, Kolling Institute, Northern Clinical School, Faculty of Medicine and Health, The University of Sydney, New South Wales, Australia

CADE Clinic, Royal North Shore Hospital, Northern Sydney Local Health District, New South Wales, Australia

Visiting Professor, Department of Psychiatry, University of Oxford, UK

Chris R. Brewin
Emeritus Professor of Psychology, Division of Psychology and Language Sciences, University College London, UK

Sally-Ann Cooper
Professor of Learning Disabilities, Institute of Health and Wellbeing, University of Glasgow, Scotland

Christopher Dowrick
Emeritus Professor of Primary Medical Care, University of Liverpool, UK

Allen Frances
Professor and Chair Emeritus, Department of Psychiatry, Duke University, Durham, North Carolina, USA

Chair, DSM-IV Task Force

Wolfgang Gaebel
Department of Psychiatry and Psychotherapy, Medical Faculty, LVR-Klinikum Düsseldorf, Heinrich-Heine-University, Düsseldorf, Germany

WHO Collaborating Centre on Quality Assurance and Empowerment in Mental Health, DEU-131, LVR-Klinikum Düsseldorf, Germany

M. Elena Garralda
Emeritus Professor of Child and Adolescent Psychiatry, Imperial College London, UK

Cary S. Kogan
Professor of Psychology, Faculty of Social Sciences, University of Ottawa, Canada

Christine Lochner
SAMRC Unit on Risk & Resilience in Mental Disorders, Dept of Psychiatry, Stellenbosch University, South Africa

Andreas Maercker
Professor and Head of the Department of Psychology, University of Zurich, Switzerland

Gin S. Malhi
Academic Department of Psychiatry, Kolling Institute, Northern Clinical School, Faculty of Medicine and Health, The University of Sydney, New South Wales, Australia

CADE Clinic, Royal North Shore Hospital, Northern Sydney Local Health District, New South Wales, Australia

Visiting Professor, Department of Psychiatry, University of Oxford, UK

Roger Mulder
Professor of Psychological Medicine, University of Otago at Christchurch, New Zealand

Geoffrey M. Reed
Professor of Medical Psychology, Department of Psychiatry, Columbia

University Vagelos College of Physicians and Surgeons

Eva Salveridou-Hof
Department of Psychiatry and Psychotherapy, Medical Faculty, LVR-Klinikum Düsseldorf, Heinrich-Heine-University, Düsseldorf, Germany

WHO Collaborating Centre on Quality Assurance and Empowerment in Mental Health, DEU-131, LVR-Klinikum Düsseldorf, Germany

John B. Saunders
National Centre for Youth Substance Use Research Faculty of Health and Behavioural Sciences, The University of Queensland, Brisbane, Queensland, Australia

Ulrike Schmidt
Professor of Eating Disorders, King's College London, UK

Dan J. Stein
SAMRC Unit on Risk & Resilience in Mental Disorders, Dept of Psychiatry and Neuroscience Institute, University of Cape Town, South Africa

Peter Tyrer
Emeritus Professor of Community Psychiatry, Imperial College London, UK

Introduction
A Guide to This Book

Peter Tyrer

Psychiatric classification is like growing old – a subject often avoided but recognized as inevitable. Whether you use a standard classification such as ICD-11 or a personal one such as 'people-I-feel-confident-in-treating' or 'people-I-prefer to avoid', it is impossible to avoid some sort of order in a subject which can present in a myriad of ways. Carl Linnaeus, not exactly a modest man, often liked to quote his prime achievement, 'God created the world, Linnaeus organized it'. His *Systema Naturae*, published in 1735, introduced the 'definitive' classification of all living organisms, organized into species, genera, classes, and orders. This classification certainly revolutionized biology and the Linnaean system continues to remain supreme, and in psychiatry we would like to aspire to a similar pinnacle of achievement if we were able to create a classification of equal standing. But please pause a minute. The Linnaean system is not definitive. Whole groups of organisms are now being refined by DNA technology and a new classification is likely to be on its way to replace or enhance it. All classifications are ephemeral.

This is a salutary lesson for all clinicians. No classification is sacrosanct, and even as we attempt to make a pale imitation of *Systema Naturae* in psychiatry[1] in creating the 11th revision of the International Classification of Diseases, we know it is bound to fail. Some critics, including a significant proportion of users of psychiatric services who have not had good experiences, wish to abandon psychiatric diagnosis in its entirety,[2] but even a modicum of thought leads to the realization that without any form of diagnosis we would turn back 400 years and allow our patients to rely only on compassion, soft words, and knowledge of the four humours in offering management.

Robert Kendell, who wrote with razor-sharp precision about psychiatric classification, once wrote, 'All our diagnostic terms are simply concepts, and the only fundamental question we can ask about them is whether they are useful concepts, and useful to whom?'[3] We must have this central element, now cast in the words 'clinical utility', repeatedly invoked in ICD-11, at the forefront of our thinking.

So we would like the reader to ask the question after reading each of the following chapters, 'Is this going to be helpful in my clinical practice?' If indeed the book does appear to be making sense by increasing understanding and promoting better practice, it will indeed represent an advance. We know already that ICD-10 did not succeed entirely in this respect. To give one example, in a Danish study of the national use of ICD-10 diagnoses, 16 diagnoses accounted for over half of all the diagnoses made for mental and behavioural disorders. These constituted only 4.2% of the 380 diagnoses available. The three most frequently registered diagnoses were paranoid schizophrenia, alcohol dependence, and adjustment disorder, used respectively in 10.2%, 8.3%, and 5.9% of the cases. At the other

1

extreme, 109 diagnoses (28.7% of all available diagnoses) were used fewer than 100 times each.[4] Put bluntly, they were either useless or, more generously, not quite fit for purpose.

This distribution would not matter if we had a high degree of certainty about our diagnostic system. A list of all the fauna in the world would show a similar distribution. But psychiatric diagnoses are not in this category. A good psychiatric diagnosis is one that conveys immediate understanding, one that is 'a clinically recognizable set of symptoms or behaviours associated in most cases with distress and with interference with personal functions'.[5] It is also paramount that any classification should be used worldwide, that it is understandable and able to be implemented in all countries, not least in those with limited resources. So, the intention is for ICD-11 to be used not only by doctors but also by other mental health professionals, other health professionals working in areas involving mental distress, and even lay health care workers.

It is also worth examining the second part of Kendell's aphorism, 'useful to whom?' If you are a counsellor in primary care or private practice seeing referrals whom you expect to treat entirely in your service, you do not need an external classification. You could make one up for yourself and signify accordingly (e.g., Type 1 problem), so when you come to see others with similar problems you can compare notes. A simple formulation at the end of the interview will normally suffice.

But when you must refer a patient to other practitioners or give a report for an external agency, you cannot rely on this approach alone. You have to use some form of communication that is relatively economical, accurate, and comprehensive. The authors of ICD-11 would like to think the revised classification will suit this demand. The World Health Organization also made it clear at the beginning of the ICD-11 classification process that its outcome should be of value in all cultures and in all countries, particularly those which have the highest burden of mental illness and the least resources.[6]

This book was created as a consequence of feedback from a two-day meeting on the 25th and 26th of May 2021 hosted by the Royal College of Psychiatrists. The 11th revision of the International Classification of Diseases has long been awaited and its publication in 2022 is thirty years after the publication of the ICD-10, a much longer period than any previous revision. The new classification is coming out at a critical time in psychiatric practice. Diagnosis in psychiatry is coming under attack on many fronts, not least from within the profession. This is partly a consequence of mistakes that have been made in the past with a superfluity of diagnoses from the introduction of DSM-III onwards. Every new diagnosis now has to be subjected to very close scrutiny and can only be introduced after a serious examination of evidence.

This is where we stumble. What is evidence for a new disorder that does not yet exist? It is almost always absent or patchy at best, and the common criticism is that the evidence gap is filled by experts who are biased in promoting their own points of view. This criticism can never be fully countered. The best we can offer is a balanced description of the advantages of the new classification over the old and a reasoned defence of the new kids on the block, with the acknowledgement that in time they will be knocked off the block in their turn.

At this stage, it is impossible to gauge whether ICD-11 will be regarded as superior to its predecessors. The maxim of Kendell's clinical utility has been adopted by the WHO in its preparation for ICD-11. This is a sensible policy, as both DSM and ICD classifications have been criticized for excessive of diagnoses ever since the success of DSM-III in 1980. It is through clinical utility that the new system will be judged.

It could be said that these changes make diagnosis fuzzier, less certain, and less crisp than formerly. But the response can be, 'Yes, maybe, but we think the changes better reflect clinical reality. Classification should be in tune with practice and if you are forced to use it because there is no alternative, something is wrong.' Anthony Storr, a psychiatrist whose writing often cut through the unnecessary verbiage of nosology, argued for a broader diagnostic approach: 'I want to show that the dividing lines between sanity and mental illness have been drawn in the wrong place. The sane are madder than we think, the mad saner' (quoted in obituary). Walled-off psychiatric diagnoses do not work.

Because we are committed to open debate, we have also invited the bête-noire of DSM-5, Allen Frances, to give his own verdict on ICD-11, especially the changes from ICD-10. We were not expecting an easy ride from Allen, and he has not pulled any punches in his criticism. Because he marshals his arguments well, they may carry conviction in some quarters. But that is for the reader to decide, and we hope that by giving alternative viewpoints each clinician can test them out in practice rather than accepting the new system as rote. The ICD-11 work groups have been examining their subjects for close on ten years; they are not, as so many believe, in hock to drug companies and corrupted by money, and no funds have been paid to them for their work. The World Health Organization has carried out this exercise on a shoestring, and throughout it has been guided by Geoffrey Reed, who has been the key to the whole enterprise.

There are many who are very keen to read the equivalent of the ICD-10 Diagnostic Guidelines published in 1993. These have moved through several names and acronyms but are now going to being published as *Clinical Descriptions and Diagnostic Requirements for ICD-11 Mental, Behavioural or Neurodevelopmental Disorders (CDDR)*.[7] These are now available from the WHO. They are not to be used for statistical recording of diagnosis but in being developed specifically for the ICD-11 Mental, Behavioural and Neurodevelopmental Disorders chapter, provide much more detailed information needed by both mental health and other health professionals to understand more fully this classification in their work with patients.

The exact text of the ICD-11 is not always replicated in this book, but it is available online – *ICD-11 who/int* then click on *ICD-11 Browser* to type in the disorder you wish to access. By giving a background to the classification rather than mere replication of the definitions, we hope that we can achieve a more sophisticated understanding of the different diagnoses.

But we are quite aware that not everything was covered at our meeting in May 2021 or in the text here. There was no presentation on eating disorders, but this has been partly compensated by Professor Ulrike Schmidt in her account of the new diagnosis of Binge-Eating Disorder. There is also no primary care version currently available, but the best available review and update is to be found in Chris Dowrick's primary care chapter at the end of the book.

Nobody at this point can say whether ICD-11 will represent a significant advance over its predecessors. This will only evolve with use over time, but our contributors have made a pretty good fist in getting the reasoning behind the changes clear for all to see.

References

1. Tyrer, P. (2013). Linnaean classification and conventional psychiatric diagnosis do not mix. *Nord J Psychiatry*, **67**, 11–12.
2. Boyle, H., Johnstone, L. (2020). *The Power Threat Meaning Framework*. Monmouth: PCCS Books.

3. Kendell, R.E. (1991). The major functional psychoses: are they independent entities or part of a continuum? In Kerr, A., McClelland, H. (Eds.), *Concepts of Mental Illness: A Continuing Debate*, pp. 1–16. London: Gaskell.

4. Munk-Jorgensen, P., Lund, M.N., Bertelsen, A. (2010). Use of ICD-10 diagnoses in Danish psychiatric hospital-based services in 2001–2007. *World Psychiatry*, **9**, 183–184.

5. World Health Organization (1992). *The ICD-10 Classification of Mental and Behavioural Disorders: Clinical Descriptions and Diagnostic Guidelines*. Geneva: World Health Organization.

6. International Advisory Group for the Revision of ICD-10 Mental and Behavioural Disorders. (2011). A conceptual framework for the revision of the ICD-10 classification of mental and behavioural disorders. *World Psychiatry*, **10**, 86–92.

7. World Health Organization (2023). *Clinical Descriptions and Diagnostic Requirements for ICD-11 Mental, Behavioural and Neurodevelopmental Disorders*. Geneva: World Health Organization.

Chapter 1

Development and Innovation in the ICD-11 Chapter on Mental, Behavioural and Neurodevelopmental Disorders

Geoffrey M. Reed

This chapter describes the context of the 11th Revision of the International Classification of Diseases (ICD-11) related to mental health. It contains an explanation of the procedure adopted in making this revision, some background to the field trials and their results, and a brief account of the main changes, many of which are amplified in the later chapters. A detailed account of the changes in the ICD-11 as compared with the ICD-10 has been published elsewhere,[1] as has a detailed comparison of the ICD-11 and the DSM-5.[2]

The context of the development of the ICD-11 is significant. This is the first major revision of the ICD in thirty years and has followed a thorough re-examination of each ICD-10 diagnosis in light of new scientific findings, best practices, and advances in information technology for health systems. The revision was approved by the World Health Assembly on 25 May 2019 and was formally implemented as a basis for health reporting by WHO member states from January 2022. Over the next few years, WHO member states will implement the ICD-11 within their clinical and health information systems. WHO has published a range of materials intended to be useful to countries in implementing the ICD-11.[3] In some systems, implementation will happen quickly and in others clinical implementation will precede full data integration. For example, Scotland has already begun the implementation of the ICD-11 classification of mental, behavioural or neurodevelopmental disorders. This will make it possible for Scottish clinicians to benefit from the more than three decades of scientific and clinical advances reflected in the ICD-11, even if their systems are still collecting data using the ICD-10 as a framework.

The Development of the ICD-11 Classification of Mental Disorders

The ICD-11 has been developed incrementally over a Fifteen-year period. The basic structure of the ICD-11 chapter on Mental, Behavioural and Neurodevelopmental Disorders (MBND) and the brief descriptions for each disorder have been online and available for review, comment, and proposals for changes[4] since 2014 (https://icd.who.int/dev11/l-m/en). The World Health Organization Department of Mental Health and Substance Use (MSD) has also developed Clinical Descriptions and Diagnostic Requirements (CDDR) for ICD-11, which are available online at https://icd.who.int/browse11/l-m/en#/ and will also be published as a book. The structure of the ICD-11 MBND classification, the category names and brief descriptions for statistical use, and the detailed diagnostic guidance for clinical implementation contained in the CDDR were developed simultaneously by seventeen expert working groups in different areas appointed by MSD. Each group included experts from all WHO regions and substantial representation of low- and middle-income countries. Working groups were responsible for reviewing the available evidence related to their areas of responsibility, including the overlapping work on the development of the DSM-5.

In making recommendations for the ICD-11, working groups were asked to consider clinical utility and global applicability[1] in addition to the validity of proposed changes. Classification is the interface between health encounters and health information. If a new diagnostic system fails to provide clinicians with enough useful information that is feasible to implement given the time and resources available to them, it is unlikely to be applied consistently and faithfully. This will have implications for the overall data used for evaluation and decision making at the system, local, national, and global levels. A more clinically useful system therefore contributes to better health data. Because of the need for global applicability, the ICD-11 MBND revision was tested via a systematic programme of global field studies. The working groups included experts from all global regions, with particular attention to the representation of low- and middle-income countries. Hundreds of global experts were involved in developing the CDDR and thousands of global clinicians were involved in testing it across the world in multiple languages, as described below.

The CDDR is designed to provide sufficient and clinically useful information to enable psychiatrists and other diagnosing health professionals to consistently and accurately apply the ICD-11 MBND classification to make diagnoses in clinical settings.[1] The sections of the CDDR follow a uniform structure,[5] which has been a major improvement over the equivalent volume for ICD-10, the Clinical Descriptions and Diagnostic Guidelines (CDDG) for ICD-10 Mental and Behavioural Disorders.[6] Each of the main disorder entries for the ICD-11 CDDR includes the following sections: 1) essential (required) features; 2) additional clinical features; 3) boundary with normality (threshold); 4) course features; 5) developmental presentations; 6) culture-related features; 7) sex and/or gender-related features; and 8) boundaries with other disorders and conditions (differential diagnosis).[5]

The essential features present briefly the characteristics of the disorder in descriptive terms.[5] They represent the clinical features that a clinician could reasonably expect to see in all cases of the disorder. In this way, they resemble diagnostic criteria in the DSM. The ICD-11 differs from the DSM-5, however, in avoiding algorithmic pseudoprecision in terms of symptom counts or precise durations unless these are well established and empirically based. (For example, in ICD-11 five of ten possible symptoms of a depressive episode must be present, one of which must be depressed mood or anhedonia; two of seven psychotic symptoms are required for a diagnosis of schizophrenia, etc.) The ICD-11 essential features are stated more flexibly than DSM-5 diagnostic criteria in order to focus on the clinical essence of the syndrome and allow sufficient room for cultural variability and informed clinical judgement to enhance global applicability. But the idea that there are no diagnostic requirements in the ICD-11 CDDR is obviously false to anyone who has actually looked at them, and it is important to stress that those making such claims are misinformed.

To take one specific example, the essential features of the ICD-11 diagnosis of PTSD can be summarized as follows[7] (see CDDR, https://icd.who.int/browse11/l-m/en#/, for the complete version):

- Exposure to an event or situation (either short- or long-lasting) of an extremely threatening or horrific nature.

- Following the traumatic event or situation, the development of a characteristic syndrome lasting for at least several weeks, consisting of three core elements:
  1. Re-experiencing the traumatic event in the present, in which the event(s) is not just remembered but is experienced as occurring again in the here and now.
  2. Deliberate avoidance of reminders likely to produce re-experiencing of the traumatic event(s).
  3. Persistent perceptions of heightened current threat.
- The disturbance causes significant impairment in functioning.

Diagnostic requirements are clearly stated, and all must be present. At the same time, the ICD-11 essential features for PTSD are vastly simpler than the diagnostic criteria in the DSM-5, which include 20 different symptoms in four different groups, as well a list of specific experiences that 'qualify' for a diagnosis that appear to be largely based on US liability concerns. It has been calculated that there are 636,120 different combinations of symptoms[8] that would qualify for a PTSD diagnosis under DSM-5.

Some have expressed concern that ICD-11's more flexible approach to diagnostic requirements would result in overdiagnosis and inflated prevalence rates, but there is no evidence to support this claim. Using World Mental Health Survey data, Stein et al.[9] found that the ICD-11 diagnostic requirements resulted in fewer diagnoses of PTSD compared with ICD-10, and comparable rates compared with DSM-5. Lago et al.[10] also applied diagnostic requirement in the major classifications to Mental Health Survey data for disorders due to use of alcohol and disorders due to use of cannabis. They found almost perfect concordance among ICD-11, DSM-IV, and ICD-10, but much lower concordance with DSM-5. Evans et al.[11] found that, compared with ICD-10 and DSM-5, the ICD-11 CDDR led to more accurate identification of severe irritability and better differentiation from boundary presentations. Participants using the DSM-5 were more likely to assign psychopathological diagnoses to developmentally normative irritability. Although relatively few head-to-head comparisons of the ICD-11 and DSM-5 have been conducted, of those that have, none has found higher rates of diagnoses using the ICD-11.

Field Testing of ICD-11 MBND

Another major area of innovation has been the extensive and systematic programme of field studies supporting the ICD-11 MBND classification and its associated CDDR.[1,12,13] Twenty internet-based case-controlled studies have been conducted using the Global Clinical Practice Network (GCPN; https://gcp.network). The GCPN is a network of over 18,500 mental health and primary care professionals from 163 countries who took part in the development of the ICD-11 through participation in field studies. Slightly more than half of GCPN members are physicians - almost all of these psychiatrists - with a third being psychologists, and the rest a mixture of other mental health disciplines. Thirty-seven per cent are working in low- and middle-income countries. GCPN studies have been conducted in a minimum of three and up to six languages: Chinese, English, French, Japanese, Russian, and Spanish. Specific studies were also conducted in German.

Case-controlled studies for ICD-11 most commonly involved participants being randomly assigned to use the ICD-11 CDDR or the ICD-10 CDDG to assign diagnoses to standardized, validated clinical case vignettes that had been manipulated to highlight key diagnostic issues.[12,13] The studies compared the accuracy and consistency of diagnostic judgements based on the two systems. Across these studies, ICD-11 consistently outperformed the ICD-10.[14,15] The methodology also permitted an examination of which specific diagnostic elements were accounting for any observed confusion, which in turn permitted refinements in the CDDR before they were finalized.[16,17]

Clinic-based studies of the reliability and clinical utility of the ICD-11 CDDR have been conducted in 14 countries covering all global regions.[18,19] These studies focused on mental disorders accounting for the greatest proportion of global disease burden and the highest levels of service utilization – schizophrenia or other primary psychotic disorders, mood disorders, anxiety or fear-related disorders, and disorders specifically associated with stress – among adult patients presenting for treatment at 29 participating centres. A concurrent joint-rater design was used, examining whether two clinicians, relying on the same clinical information, agreed on the diagnosis when separately applying the ICD-11 CDDR. Intraclass kappa coefficients for diagnoses weighted by site and study prevalence ranged from 0.45 (dysthymic disorder) to 0.88 (social anxiety disorder) and would be considered moderate to almost perfect for all diagnoses.[17] Overall, the reliability of the ICD-11 CDDR was superior to that previously reported for equivalent ICD-10 guidelines. Clinician ratings of the clinical utility of the proposed ICD-11 diagnostic guidelines were very positive overall.[18] The CDDR were perceived as easy to use, corresponding accurately to patients' presentations (i.e., goodness of fit), clear and understandable, providing an appropriate level of detail, taking about the same or less time than clinicians' usual practice, and providing useful guidance about distinguishing disorder from normality and from other disorders.

The reliability results from the clinic-based studies challenge the claim that some have put forward that the more clinician-friendly, less concretely algorithmic, and less highly operationalized approach adopted for the ICD-11 CDDR is inherently less reliable. The concern that the ICD-11 CDDR has sacrificed reliability is not based on any data, but rather based on assumptions that have been built into the DSM since DSM-III, including the assumptions that clinicians apply the criteria as they are written, which we do not believe is the case. In our clinic-based studies, clinicians with diverse training and experience used the ICD-11 CDDR following a relatively brief training (about 4 hours) to conduct routine clinical assessments (lasting about 1 hour) using open form interviews. They obtained reliability coefficients similar to those achieved using more complex and time-consuming structured instruments.[19–21] It is possible that further gains in reliability among clinicians could be obtained by focusing greater attention on appropriate training in diagnostic skills and interviewing techniques, rather than on continuing to devote attention and resources to introducing greater precision in operationalization as a part of successive refinements in diagnostic criteria.

New Disorder Categories

Twenty-three new disorders have been added to the ICD-11 MBND chapter (see Table 1.1), reflecting either a distinct disorder that was not classifiable in the ICD-10 (e.g., Hoarding Disorder), or a disorder that is a result of extending, expanding, or subdividing an existing disorder in such a way that has resulted in a new disorder rather than a subtype (e.g., Binge Eating Disorder).[22] Most of these were either already in the DSM-IV or added to the DSM-5.

Table 1.1 New categories in the ICD-11 chapter on mental, behavioural, or neurodevelopmental disorders

Disorder grouping	New disorder
Catatonia	Catatonia (previously a subtype of schizophrenia)
Mood disorders	Bipolar type II disorder (previously included in bipolar affective disorder)
Obsessive–compulsive or related disorders	Body dysmorphic disorder Olfactory reference disorder Hoarding disorder Excoriation (skin picking) disorder
Disorders specifically associated with stress	Complex post-traumatic stress disorder Prolonged grief disorder
Dissociative disorders	Partial dissociative identity disorder
Feeding or eating disorders	Binge eating disorder Avoidant–restrictive food intake disorder Rumination–regurgitation disorder
Disorder of bodily distress or bodily experience	Body integrity dysphoria
Disorders due to substance use or addictive behaviours	Substance-induced anxiety disorder Substance-induced obsessive-compulsive or related disorder Substance-induced impulse control disorder Gaming disorder
Impulse control disorders	Compulsive sexual behaviour disorder Intermittent explosive disorder
Factitious disorders	Factitious disorder imposed on another
Secondary mental or behavioural syndromes associated with disorders or diseases classified elsewhere	Secondary neurodevelopmental syndrome Secondary obsessive-compulsive or related syndrome Secondary impulse control syndrome

The effect of adding these categories has therefore generally been to enhance compatibility between the ICD-11 and the DSM-5.

The most consequential additions are arguably four new disorders in the ICD-11 that represent different decisions than were taken for the DSM-5. These are Complex PTSD, Prolonged Grief Disorder, Gaming Disorder, and Compulsive Sexual Behaviour Disorder, although Prolonged Grief Disorder has since been added to the DSM 5.1 and Internet Gaming Disorder appears in the DSM-5 and DSM 5.1 research appendix. We have published a detailed review of the rationale and consequences of adding these four disorders,[22] concluding that each describes an important and distinctive clinical population that is an appropriate focus of health services and with specific treatment needs that would otherwise likely go unmet. WHO's announced intention to include these categories has clearly facilitated an expansion of research in each area, which has generally supported their validity and utility, as well as increased availability of appropriate services.

Complex PTSD

The essential or required features of complex PTSD include all three core symptoms of PTSD (re-experiencing in the present, avoidance, and ongoing sense of threat). Additional features of complex PTSD include three characteristic types of disturbances in self-organization: severe and persistent problems in affect regulation; beliefs about the self as diminished, defeated, or worthless; and difficulties in sustaining relationships and in feeling close to others.[7,22] Complex PTSD is more likely to be the product of certain types of traumas, such as prolonged or repetitive events from which escape is difficult or impossible (e.g., torture, slavery, prolonged domestic violence, repeated childhood sexual or physical abuse), and typically requires longer and more complex treatments than does PTSD. However, treatments for complex PTSD are not typically as long or as complex as evidence-based treatments for borderline personality disorder. Emerging evidence indicates that complex PTSD and borderline personality disorder are quite distinct, having only the feature of affect dysregulation in common.[22-24]

Prolonged Grief Disorder

The essential features of prolonged grief disorder include persistent longing or yearning for the deceased and associated intense emotional pain, difficulty accepting the death, a feeling of having lost a part of oneself, an inability to experience positive mood, emotional numbing, and difficulty in engaging with social or other activities.[7,22] The severe grief response needs to persist beyond 6 months after bereavement, or for a time that clearly exceeds the norms of the person's culture, and produce significant impairment in personal, social, or occupational functioning.

There has been accumulating evidence over many years that supports prolonged grief disorder as a specific and identifiable condition that can severely impact a minority of bereaved people.[22] This is not to say that the experience and expression of grief, bereavement, and mourning are not deeply personal and individual. The CDDR also attend carefully to cultural variation in mourning customs and duration. At the same time, for individuals who continue to experience constant and intense emotional pain that interferes with their ability to function 6 months or more following the death, convergent evidence from multiple controlled trials indicates that grief-focused psychotherapy is effective in alleviating their suffering.[25] This treatment is specific to prolonged grief disorder and distinct from interventions for depression. A more standardized approach to diagnosing prolonged grief disorder in the CDDR can therefore be helpful in directing persons with this condition to the best available care.

Gaming Disorder

In the ICD-11, gaming disorder is characterized by a pattern of persistent or recurrent gaming behaviour ('digital gaming' or 'video-gaming'), manifested by:

1. impaired control over gaming (e.g., onset, frequency, intensity, duration, termination, context);
2. increasing priority given to gaming to the extent that gaming takes precedence over other life interests and daily activities; and
3. continuation or escalation of gaming despite the occurrence of negative consequences.

The pattern of gaming behaviour results in marked distress or significant impairment in personal, family, social, educational, occupational, or other important areas of functioning. The gaming behaviour and other features are normally evident over a period of at least 12 months in order for a diagnosis to be assigned.[22,26]

The CDDR for gaming disorder are particularly careful to distinguish it from non-pathological involvement in gaming activities. An international Delphi study[27] examined the validity, clinical utility, and prognostic value of the proposed ICD-11 diagnostic requirements, as well as the DSM-5 research criteria for Internet gaming disorder. Participating experts agreed that the ICD-11 CDDR were likely to identify the condition adequately, and more like'ly to avoid pathologizing intensive but non-pathological gaming behaviours. The global gaming industry has vigorously opposed the inclusion of gaming disorder in the ICD-11,[28,29] and has promoted scholars who challenge the disorder and direct public attention to research highlighting the benefits of gaming.

Compulsive Sexual Behaviour Disorder

In the ICD-11, compulsive sexual behaviour disorder is characterized by a persistent pattern of failure to control intense, repetitive sexual impulses or urges resulting in repetitive sexual behaviour over an extended period (6 months or more). Symptoms may include repetitive sexual activities becoming a central focus of the person's life to the point of neglecting health and personal care or other interests, activities, and responsibilities; numerous unsuccessful efforts to significantly reduce repetitive sexual behaviour; and continued repetitive sexual behaviour despite adverse consequences or deriving little or no satisfaction from it. The symptoms cause marked distress or significant impairment in personal, family, social, educational, occupational, or other important areas of functioning.[22,30]

The ICD-11 CDDR make extremely clear that distress related to moral judgements and disapproval about sexual impulses, urges, or behaviours is not sufficient to meet this requirement. The CDDR also carefully address concerns about false positives and the stigmatization of non-pathological sexual behaviour, alerting that particular attention must be paid to the evaluation of individuals who self-identify as having the condition (e.g., calling themselves 'sex addicts' or 'porn addicts') to verify that they actually exhibit the clinical characteristics of the disorder. There has been discussion about whether such a disorder should more appropriately be regarded as a behavioural addiction.[31] ICD-11 adopted a more cautious policy of including it in the grouping of impulse control disorders and separating it from the addictions in the light of some differences from substance use disorders, gambling, and gaming disorder.[32]

Mental Disorder Categories That Have Been Removed from the ICD-11

Those who express concern about the ever-expanding encroachment of psychiatric disorder categories on everyday life may be reassured to learn that an even greater number of mental disorder categories have been removed from the ICD-11 than have been added. The new dimensional diagnostic systems for schizophrenia or other primary psychotic disorders and for personality disorders described in later chapters in this book mean that the subtypes of schizophrenia and the specific personality disorders in the ICD-10 are no longer part of the classification. Detailed subtypes of acute and transient psychotic disorder and adjustment disorder are no longer included in the ICD-11. A number of 'mixed' disorders, particularly in categories describing children and adolescents, have been removed (e.g., hyperactive conduct disorder, depressive conduct disorder). Separate categories for childhood-specific forms of anxiety disorder have been dropped and are rather described as developmental presentations in the main classification of anxiety or fear-related disorders. Categories that in the ICD-10 were designed to be assigned based on a homosexual or bisexual orientation (i.e., sexual maturation disorder, egodystonic sexual orientation, sexual relationship disorder) have been eliminated.[33]

Other Innovations in ICD-11 MBND

Several other innovations in the ICD-11 bear emphasis here. First, the ICD-11 has largely eliminated the 'mind–body split' that was inherent in the ICD-10 classification of mental disorders. In ICD-10, a distinction was made between 'organic' and 'non-organic' forms of cognitive disorders, sleep disorders, and sexual dysfunctions. This separation is inconsistent with our current understanding of the development and maintenance of these disorders. The ICD-11 contains a new, unified classification of sexual dysfunctions in the new chapter on Conditions Related to Sexual Health, which integrates categories previously classified as mental disorders with others that were classified primarily as diseases of the genitourinary system. Similarly, a new chapter on Sleep–Wake Disorders integrates sleep disorders previously classified as mental disorders, diseases of the nervous system, and diseases of the respiratory system. A unified syndromal description of dementia and other neurocognitive disorders, including different levels of severity and categories describing behavioural and psychological disturbances in dementia, is provided in the MBND chapter of the ICD-11. These categories can be linked to categories indicating underlying causes (e.g., diseases of the nervous system, infectious diseases, substance use disorders).

Another innovation is the integration of dimensional approaches within the categorical structure of ICD-11. There has been increasing recognition over the past 40 years that most mental and behavioural disorders are best thought of as representing several underlying dimensions rather than discrete categories.[34] The ICD is fundamentally a categorical system with specific nosological and formal requirements, and there are many clinical, scientific, and practical benefits to the inclusion of mental disorders alongside other classes of diseases as part of the ICD-11.[35] The ICD-11 has introduced a range of important structural innovations based on a transition to a fully electronic system, which has made it possible to integrate substantial dimensional information within the ICD's categorical approach. The dimensional potential of the ICD-11 has been most fully realized in the areas of schizophrenia and other primary psychotic disorders[36] as well as personality disorders.[37,38] These innovations are fully described in other chapters of this book. Overall, the dimensional approach puts a stronger focus on the current presentation and therefore treatment needs in the present, rather than emphasizing a diagnosis as something that signifies a characteristic of the person that is stable over time. This is more consistent with a recovery-based approach and makes it possible to document improvements in clinical presentation that do not necessarily alter the underlying diagnosis.

The classification of disorders due to substance use has also been changed substantially in response to global public health needs.[39] The range of substance classes has been updated and expanded in response to diversification of psychoactive substances and changes in their routes of administration and the contexts of their use, including the rapid development and diffusion of new, synthetic psychoactive substances. The ICD-11 has retained the concept of harmful use of psychoactive substances, that is, patterns of substance use that cause significant harm to physical or mental health, because of its public health importance and the opportunities it provides for intervention in primary care and other non-specialist settings. Different patterns of harmful use have been specified, including a new category for single episodes as well as episodic or continuous patterns of use. Harm to others as a result of substance use has been newly incorporated into the CDDR in the section on harmful use. The diagnostic requirements for substance dependence have been reformulated so they can more easily be identified in a variety of settings. These changes present significant opportunities for prevention, treatment, and health policy at a variety of levels.

Finally, major changes have been made in the classification of gender identity in ICD-11, based on advances in research and clinical practice, and major shifts in social attitudes and in relevant policies, laws, and human rights standards.[40] What were called gender identity disorders in ICD-11 have been reconceptualized as gender incongruence and moved to the new ICD-11 chapter on Conditions Related to Sexual Health. That is, WHO no longer considers the experience of having a transgender identity to be a mental disorder. This change was supported by a programme of research indicating that distress and functional impairment among transgender people are strongly related to experiences of stigmatization and victimization rather than being an inherent aspect of being transgender.[41,42] The categories were not removed from ICD-11 altogether because they were seen as important in many countries in securing access to gender-affirming services.[43]

Next Steps

The ICD-11 will be implemented around the world during the next several years. WHO is actively working with member states on implementation, and the Department of Mental Health and Substance Use has established an Advisory Group for Training and Implementation of ICD-11 Mental, Behavioural, or Neurodevelopmental Disorder, including experts from all global regions as well as government health officials directly involved in implementation at the country level.

In addition, there is a huge need for psychiatrists, psychologists, and other mental health professionals to be trained in how to use ICD-11 in clinical settings. WHO has been actively collaborating with professional societies including the Royal College of Psychiatrists in advancing this agenda. A detailed online training programme consisting of 15 training units, each focusing on a major grouping of disorders, has been developed and is currently available in English (https://gmhacademy.dialogedu.com) and Spanish (https://gmhacademy.dialogedu.com/cie-11). Other resources are available to members of the Global Clinical Practice Network (visit https://gcp.network/ to register). We hope that this book will be an important part of ICD-11 dissemination and training and that it will be useful to psychiatrists and other health professionals providing services to people with mental disorders around the world.

References

1. Reed, G.M., First, M.B., Kogan, C.S., et al. (2019). Innovations and changes in the ICD-11 classification of mental, behavioural and neurodevelopmental disorders. *World Psychiatry*, **18**(1), 3–19. https://doi.org/10.1002/wps.20611

2. First, M.B., Gaebel, W., Maj, M., et al. (2021). An organization- and category-level comparison of diagnostic requirements for mental disorders in ICD-11 and DSM-5. *World Psychiatry*, **20**(1), 34–51. https://doi.org/10.1002/wps.20825

3. World Health Organization. (2019). ICD-11 Implementation or Transition Guide. Geneva: World Health Organization. https://doi.org//icd.who.int/docs/ICD-11%20Implementation%20or%20Transition%20Guide_v105.pdf
4. Fuss, J., Lemay, K., Stein, D.J., et al. (2019). Public stakeholders' comments on ICD-11 chapters related to mental and sexual health. *World Psychiatry*, **18**, 233–235.
5. First, M.B., Reed, GM., Hyman, S.E., Saxena, S. (2015). The development of the ICD-11 Clinical Descriptions and Diagnostic Guidelines for Mental and Behavioural Disorders. *World Psychiatry*, **14**(1), 82–90. https://doi.org/10.1002/wps.20189
6. World Health Organization. (1992). *The ICD-10 Classification of Mental and Behavioural Disorders: Clinical Descriptions and Diagnostic Guidelines*. Geneva: World Health Organization.
7. Maercker, A., Brewin, C.R., Bryant, R.A., et al. (2013). Diagnosis and classification of disorders specifically associated with stress: proposals for ICD-11. *World Psychiatry*, **12**, 198–206.
8. Galatzer-Levy, I.R. & Bryant, R.A. (2013). 636,120 ways to have posttraumatic stress disorder. *Perspect Psychol Sci*, **8**, 651–662.
9. Stein, D.J., McLaughlin, K.A., Koenen, K.C., et al. (2014). DSM-5 and ICD-11 definitions of posttraumatic stress disorder: investigating 'narrow' and 'broad' approaches. *Depress Anxiety*, **31**, 494–505.
10. Lago, L., Bruno, R., Degenhardt, L. (2016). Concordance of ICD-11 and DSM-5 definitions of alcohol and cannabis use disorders: a population survey. *Lancet Psychiatry*, **3**(7), 673–684. https://doi.org/10.1016/S2215-0366(16)00088-2
11. Evans, S.C., Roberts, M.C., Keeley, J.W., et al. (2021). Diagnostic classification of irritability and oppositionality in youth: a global field study comparing ICD-11 with ICD-10 and DSM-5. *J Child Psychol Psychiatry*, **62**, 303–312.
12. Keeley, J.W., Reed, G.M., Roberts, M.C., et al. (2016). Developing a science of clinical utility in diagnostic classification systems: field study strategies for ICD-11 Mental and Behavioural Disorders. *Am Psychol*, **71**, 3–16.
13. Evans, S.C., Roberts, M.C., Keeley, J.W., et al. (2015). Vignette methodologies for studying clinicians' decision-making: validity, utility, and application in field studies for ICD-11. *Int J Clin Health Psychol*, **15**, 160–170.
14. Claudino, A.M., Pike, K.M., Hay, P., et al. (2019). The classification of feeding and eating disorders in the ICD-11: results of a field study comparing proposed ICD-11 guidelines with existing ICD-10 guidelines. *BMC Med*, **17**, 93.
15. Kogan, C.S., Stein, D.J., Rebello, T.J., et al. (2020). Accuracy of diagnostic judgments using ICD-11 vs. ICD-10 diagnostic guidelines for obsessive-compulsive and related disorders. *J Affect Disord*, **273**, 328–340.
16. Keeley, J.W., Reed, G.M., Roberts, M.C., et al. (2016). Disorders specifically associated with stress: a case-controlled field study for ICD-11 Mental and Behavioural Disorders. *Int J Clin Health Psychol*, **16**, 109–127.
17. Reed, G.M., Sharan, P., Rebello, T.J., et al. (2018). The ICD-11 developmental field study of reliability of diagnoses of high-burden mental disorders: results among adult patients in mental health settings of 13 countries. *World Psychiatry*, **17**, 174–186.
18. Reed, G.M., Sharan, P., Rebello, T.J., et al. (2018). Clinical utility of ICD-11 diagnostic guidelines for high-burden mental disorders: results from mental health settings in 13 countries. *World Psychiatry*, **17**, 306–315.
19. Chmielewski, M., Clark, L.A., Bagby R.M., et al. (2015). Method matters: understanding diagnostic reliability in DSM-IV and DSM-5. *J Abnorm Psychol*, **124**, 764–769.
20. Andrews, G., Peters, L., Guzman, A-M., et al. (1995). A comparison of two structured diagnostic interviews: CIDI and SCAN. *Aust N Z J Psychiatry*, **29**, 124–132.
21. Lobbestael, J., Leurgans, M., Arntz, A. (2011). Inter-rater reliability of the

Structured Clinical Interview for DSM-IV Axis I Disorders (SCID I) and Axis II Disorders (SCID II). *Clin Psychol Psychother*, **18**, 75–79.

22. Reed, G.M., First, M.B., Billieux, J., et al. (2022). Emerging experience with selected new categories in the ICD-11: complex PTSD, prolonged grief disorder, gaming disorder, and compulsive sexual behaviour disorder. *World Psychiatry*, **21**(2), 189–213. https://doi.org/10.1002/wps.20960

23. Hyland, P., Karatzias, T., Shevlin, M., et al. (2019). Examining the discriminant validity of complex posttraumatic stress disorder and borderline personality disorder symptoms: results from a United Kingdom population sample. *J Trauma Stress*, **32**, 855–863.

24. Frost, R., Murphy, J., Hyland, P., et al. (2020). Revealing what is distinct by recognising what is common: distinguishing between complex PTSD and Borderline Personality Disorder symptoms using bifactor modelling. *Eur J Psychotraumatol*, **11**, 1836864.

25. Bryant, R.A., Kenny, L., Joscelyne, A., et al. (2014). Treating prolonged grief disorder: a randomized controlled trial. *JAMA Psychiatry*, **71**, 1332–9.

26. Rumpf, H.J., Achab, S., Billieux, J., et al. (2018). Including gaming disorder in the ICD-11: the need to do so from a clinical and public health perspective. *J Behav Addict*, **7**(3), 556–561. https://doi.org/10.1556/2006.7.2018.59

27. Castro-Calvo, J., King, D.L., Stein, D.J., et al. (2021). Expert appraisal of criteria for assessing gaming disorder: an international Delphi study. *Addiction*, **116**(9), 2463–2475. https://doi.org/10.1111/add.15411

28. King, D.L.; Gaming Industry Response Consortium. (2018). Comment on the global gaming industry's statement on ICD-11 gaming disorder: a corporate strategy to disregard harm and deflect social responsibility? *Addiction*, **113**, 2145–2146.

29. European Games Developer Foundation. (2018). Statement on WHO ICD-11 list and the inclusion of gaming. www.egdf.eu.

30. Kraus, S.W., Krueger, R.B., Briken, P., et al. (2018). Compulsive sexual behaviour disorder in the ICD-11. *World Psychiatry*, **17**(1), 109–110. https://doi.org/10.1002/wps.20499

31. Kraus, S.W., Voon, V., Potenza, M.N. (2016). Should compulsive sexual behavior be considered an addiction? *Addiction*, **111**, 2097–2106.

32. Stein, D.J., Billieux, J., Bowden-Jones, H., et al. (2018). Balancing validity, utility and public health considerations in disorders due to addictive behaviours. *World Psychiatry*, **17**(3), 363–364. https://doi.org/10.1002/wps.20570

33. Cochran, S.D., Drescher, J., Kismödi, E., et al. (2014). Proposed declassification of disease categories related to sexual orientation in the International Statistical Classification of Diseases and Related Health Problems (ICD-11). *Bull World Health Organ*, **92**, 672–679. https://doi.org/10.2471/BLT.14.135541

34. Clark, L.A., Cuthbert, B., Lewis-Fernández, R., Narrow, W., Reed, G.M. (2017). ICD-11, DSM-5, and RDoC: three approaches to understanding and classifying mental disorder. *PSPI*, **18**, 72–145.

35. International Advisory Group for the Revision of ICD-10 Mental and Behavioural Disorders. (2011). A conceptual framework for the revision of the ICD-10 classification of mental and behavioural disorders. *World Psychiatry*, **10**(2), 86–92. https://doi.org/.1002/j.2051-5545.2011.tb00022.xUnlinked

36. Gaebel, W. (2012). Status of psychotic disorders in ICD-11 [published correction appears in Schizophr Bull. 2012 Nov;38(6), 1336]. *Schizophr Bull*, **38**(5), 895–898. https://doi.org/10.1093/schbul/sbs104

37. Tyrer, P., Crawford, M., Mulder, R.; ICD-11 Working Group for the Revision of Classification of Personality Disorders. (2011). Reclassifying personality disorders. *Lancet*, **377**(9780), 1814–1815. https://doi.org/10.1016/S0140-6736(10)61926-5

38. Reed, G.M. (2018). Progress in developing a classification of personality

39. Poznyak, V., Reed, G.M., Medina-Mora, M.E. (2018). Aligning the ICD-11 classification of disorders due to substance use with global service needs. *Epidemiol Psychiatr Sci*, **27**(3), 212–218. https://doi.org/10.1017/S2045796017000622

40. Reed, G.M., Drescher, J., Krueger, R.B., et al. (2016). Disorders related to sexuality and gender identity in the ICD-11: revising the ICD-10 classification based on current scientific evidence, best clinical practices, and human rights considerations. *World Psychiatry*, **15**, 205–221.

disorders for ICD-11. *World Psychiatry*, **17**(2), 227–229. https://doi.org/10.1002/wps.20533

41. Robles, R., Fresán, A., Vega-Ramírez, H., et al. (2016). Removing transgender identity from the classification of mental disorders: a Mexican field study for ICD-11. *Lancet Psychiatry*, **3**, 850–859.

42. Robles, R., Keeley, J.W., Vega-Ramírez, H., et al. (2022). Validity of categories related to gender identity in ICD-11 and DSM-5 among transgender individuals who seek gender-affirming medical procedures. *Int J Clin Health Psychol*, **22**(1), 100281. https://doi.org/10.1016/j.ijchp.2021.100281

43. Drescher, J., Cohen-Kettenis, P., Winter, S. (2012). Minding the body: situating gender identity diagnoses in the ICD-11. *Int Rev Psychiatry*, **24**(6), 568–577. https://doi.org/10.3109/09540261.2012.741575

Chapter 2

ICD-11 + DSM-5 = A Diagnostic Babel

Allen Frances

Let us confuse their language so they will not understand each other.
Genesis 11:7

The ICD and DSM are both useful systems of psychiatric diagnosis, alike enough to be roughly comparable, but different enough to cause confusion and misuse. Both systems are in wide use around the world and are likely to remain so. Neither system is clearly better than the other – we would be much better off having either one, rather than both.

The ICD-11 and DSM-5 also share the same major flaws. Both provide very loose definitions of 'mental disorder' that encourage the overdiagnosis of people with minor problems and the neglect of those with severe ones. Both are based mostly on the consensus of experts who were strongly biased towards adding new diagnoses. Neither required the presence of compelling scientific evidence to support adding new diagnoses or making changes in existing ones.

One of my main goals for DSM-IV 30 years ago was to reduce disparities between it and ICD-10 (which was prepared at the same time). We convened numerous meetings, bringing together teams of experts working on both systems, hoping to forge mutually acceptable compromise definitions for as many disorders as possible. Sometimes we succeeded, but mostly we failed. Local preferences, professional rivalries, and national loyalties tended to trump ecumenical cooperation. The separate groups that later created DSM-5 and ICD-11 have unfortunately widened the gulf even further between the two systems.

I will discuss eleven of the new disorders that were newly added to ICD-11. Some of these had already been introduced by DSM-IV (Bipolar II) or DSM-5 (Catatonia; Binge Eating; Premenstrual Dysphoric; Hoarding); some were given official recognition for the first time in ICD-11 (Complex PTSD; Prolonged Grief; Gaming; Compulsive Sexual Behaviour; Body Integrity Dysphoria; and a radically new system of diagnosing Personality Disorder).

Why so many new diagnoses in ICD-11? Unfortunately, it failed to learn from DSM-5's mistakes and made no effort to contain the ever-exploding inflation in psychiatric diagnosis. Both systems gave their expert consultants far too much control over final decision making. Experts in each area of psychiatric diagnosis are necessary contributors to the process of revising the diagnostic system – but they should never be allowed final decision-making power over their own area of particular interest. Experts always love their research pets, hype their benefits, ignore their risks. They worry greatly about missed patients, while blithely ignoring the risks of mislabelling normals. New diagnoses that work for experts in hothouse research environments are often a disaster in real-world psychiatric and primary care practice. I have never known any experts, among the many hundreds I've worked with, to ever suggest narrowing the definitions in their area of expertise. Their bias is always to accept new diagnoses and loosen definitional thresholds for existing ones.

Adding new diagnoses almost always turns out to be a bad idea – achieving smaller than expected benefits and risking harmful unrecognized and unintended consequences. Most seemingly promising contenders wind up causing far more problems than they solve. We were very cautious about adding new diagnoses in DSM-IV and accepted only two from among the ninety-four suggested. Both (Bipolar II and Asperger's) had compelling rationales; extensive literatures; thorough field testing; universal consent. Nonetheless, both triggered unexpected fads of excessive diagnosis and both probably did much more harm than good by virtue of their unanticipated, harmful, unintended consequences. The DSM-5 and ICD-11 have been remarkably welcoming of new diagnoses; they required little empirical support; did little field testing; and fearlessly and carelessly expanded already existing diagnostic inflation.

Overdiagnosis is also encouraged by another new feature of ICD-11. Although it contains criteria sets that look like those in DSM-5, ICD-11 does not offer thresholds for the number of symptoms required before making a diagnosis. Clinicians are instead permitted to use their own clinical judgement when deciding how closely any given patient meets the prototype provided for a given disorder. This makes ICD-11 much easier to use by busy practitioners, but also inherently unreliable and essentially useless for research. It also means that patients on the fuzzy boundary between normal and disorder are more likely to be diagnosed as disordered rather than regarded as subclinical.

By virtue of its many new diagnoses and its abolition of required symptom thresholds, ICD-11 has become the most overinclusive of all the diagnostic systems ever produced in the history of psychiatry. Any future increases in the reported rates of psychiatric disorder should be attributed to the changes ICD-11 has made in the diagnostic system – not to human nature suddenly getting sicker. Tens (or perhaps hundreds) of millions of people around the world who would have been considered normal using previous diagnostic systems will now qualify for an ICD-11 diagnosis.

Disorders Rejected by DSM-5 but Included in ICD-11

The DSM-5 Task Force displayed a strong and consistent bias towards introducing new disorders – consistently exaggerating potential benefits while neglecting very real risks. Published 6 years later, ICD-11 might have learned from DSM-5's overinclusiveness – but did not. Instead of avoiding further diagnostic inflation, ICD-11 was reckless enough to accept as official categories a large number of new disorders so clearly unworthy they had been roundly rejected by DSM-5. (Editor's note: in Chapter 1, Geoffrey Reed states that more disorders were removed in ICD-11 than added.)

'Prolonged Grief Disorder'

There can never be a uniform expiration date on normal grief – and ICD-11 should not have felt empowered to impose one. People grieve in their own ways, for periods of time that vary widely depending on the person; the nature of the loss; and relevant cultural practices. Mislabelling grief as mental disorder stigmatizes the grievers; exposes them to unneeded psychiatric medication; and insults the dignity of their loss. The decision to declare 'Prolonged Grief' a psychiatric disorder was based on minimal research by just a few research teams; has not been field tested in a wide array of practice settings to smoke out harmful unintended consequences; and, perhaps most importantly, creates many new problems while serving no useful purpose. If a diagnosis is needed for prolonged grievers suffering 'clinically significant distress or impairment', 'Major Depressive Disorder' or 'Adjustment Disorder' have always been available and should be used now. I strongly encourage clinicians to use common sense and clinical judgement. Don't follow any ICD-11-induced fad to suddenly pathologize what is one of humanity's most ubiquitous, basic, and essential life experiences.

'Complex PTSD'

The ICD-11 provides a very narrow definition for its new diagnosis 'Complex PTSD'. The patient must meet all criteria for PTSD and in addition have 'persistent, pervasive, and enduring disturbances in affect regulation, self-concept, and relational functioning'. These symptoms were previously covered in DSM-5 and ICD-10 as associated features of PTSD. I see no great gain in creating this entirely new PTSD diagnosis just to describe its most severe and persistent form. And there is one potential great harm – ICD-11's narrow 'Complex PTSD' may be confused with a much broader and much riskier conception of 'Complex PTSD' that was rightfully rejected by both DSM-IV and DSM-5. The label 'Complex PTSD', as it was proposed for DSM and as it is commonly used in the literature, dramatically loosens the 'PTSD' definition by including many of the most common problems adults present with and attributing them to a wide array of often poorly defined and hard to determine childhood traumas. The DSM proposals were wildly overinclusive and impossibly unreliable, and made the bold claim that much of adult psychopathology is caused by childhood trauma. Symptoms were non-specific, far ranging, and overlapping with many other disorders, including shame, guilt, anxiety, difficulty in controlling emotions, impulsivity, dissociation, persistent physical symptoms, interpersonal problems, self-destructive and suicidal behaviours, substance abuse, and personality problems. To avoid possible confusion between the narrow ICD-11 definition and common usage, I suggest clinicians avoid the diagnosis 'Complex PTSD' and instead use 'PTSD, severe'.

'Behavioural Addictions'

The ICD-11 has added two new 'behavioural addictions' ('Gaming Disorder' and 'Compulsive Sexual Behaviour Disorder') to the one already included in DSM-5 ('Gambling Disorder'). This is a risky and slippery slope – behavioural addictions could eventually be easily expanded to include passionate attachments to many other common activities – shopping, exercise, work, golf, sunbathing, model railroading, and – you name it. All passionate interests are at risk for redefinition as mental disorders. It is extremely difficult to distinguish the relatively few people who are really enslaved by gambling, gaming, or sex from the huge army of those who are attached to these pleasurable activities as normal recreation. Behaviours should not be counted as mental disorders just because people derive a lot of pleasure from them and devote much time to them. Addiction requires that the person be compulsively stuck doing something that's no longer fun, feels out of control, serves no useful purpose, and is certainly not worth the pain, costs, and harms. The unfavourable cost/benefit ratio must be pretty lopsided before mental disorder is considered. We all do foolish things that offer short-term pleasures but cause bad long-term consequences. That's our human nature – derived from many millions of years of evolutionary experience where life was short, opportunities for pleasure rare, and the long term didn't count for nearly as much as it does now.

Gaming Disorder

I opposed the inclusion of Gaming Disorder in DSM-5, but have since changed my mind and now approve its inclusion in ICD-11. Circumstances have changed a great deal in the intervening decade. Compulsive gaming is becoming both increasingly common and much more destructive – in some countries, it is the cause of severe, sometimes total, social withdrawal among a substantial number of people, especially the young. Computer games become more dangerous as they become more compelling – virtual reality replacing the real reality of school, work, family, friends, romantic relationships, even eating and sleeping. Gaming Disorder should not be used lightly to mislabel people who just like gaming but have it under control. The person who qualifies for the diagnosis must show signs of 1) tolerance – needing more to get the same kick; 2) withdrawal – feeling terrible when trying to stop; and 3) a pattern of compulsive use – continuing to play even if the pleasure is largely gone and the cost is extremely high (e.g., terrible work, interpersonal, financial, health, and/or legal consequences).

Gaming Disorder will lose its value as a diagnosis if it is trivialized by careless misapplication to everyone who just likes to play a lot but is not much harmed by it.

Compulsive Sexual Behaviour Disorder

Despite its bias to carelessly include new diagnoses, DSM-5 wisely excluded proposals for 'compulsive sexuality' or 'hypersexuality'. These were snubbed due to the lack of research, loose definitions, and high levels of potential for misuse. It doesn't make sense to risk mislabelling the vast majority of sexual miscreants as 'mentally disordered' in order to capture the very few who are truly compulsive. A broadened and cheapened concept of behavioural addiction weakens personal accountability. 'Sorry honey [or Judge], my sex addiction made me do it.' ICD-11 threw this rare example of DSM-5 caution to the wind. Its new category 'Compulsive Sexual Behaviour Disorder' may be appropriate for the very small few whose troubling sexual behaviours are truly compulsive, but it is likely to be misapplied to many who are merely impulsive and irresponsible.

Body Integrity Dysphoria

Body Integrity Dysphoria describes patients who renounce a healthy limb and often request it be amputated. The diagnosis was first proposed in 1977; has been reported in only about 100 patients; has been studied by only a few research groups; has no treatment; and may belong more within the realm of neurology than psychiatry. Despite all these cautionary signs, Body Integrity Dysphoria was included in ICD-11 because one of the ICD-11 leaders has also been the major contributor to its meagre literature. This is the clearest possible example of an expert having excessive influence on the diagnostic system. Including Body Identity Dysphoria in ICD-11 is also not without considerable risks. Its premature legitimization as an official category will undoubtedly be used to justify maiming surgeries and may potentially trigger a fad of copycat symptom presentations.

Personality Disorder

Personality Disorder diagnosis reached its greatest prominence in 1980 when it was given its own axis in the five-axis 'Multiaxial System' of DSM-III. Each diagnostic evaluation was meant to consider the important, but routinely neglected, question of whether personality disorder was also present or absent, independent of the diagnosis of other DSM disorders. This is highly desirable because personality disorder is sometimes the main target of treatment and often an important factor in treatment selection and successful outcome, whatever may be the primary diagnosis. When DSM-5 unwisely eliminated the 'Multiaxial System', personality disorders were demoted to just another category and were most often neglected. The ICD-11 completes the marginalization of personality diagnosis by introducing a completely new system that will likely be used rarely, if at all.

The ICD-11 meant well. Everyone knows that personality disorders do not have sharp boundaries from normality; from other psychiatric disorders; and from adjustment disorders caused by severe and prolonged real-life stressors. It is also well known that dimensional rating is much more accurate than categorical naming in describing continuous variables like personality. I wrote the last draft of the DSM-III Personality Disorders section in 1980, but simultaneously also suggested in papers and talks that it should eventually be replaced by a dimensional format. In preparing DSM-IV, we tried, but failed, to forge agreement among proponents of the various dimensional systems. We dropped the effort, but I wrote a paper called 'Dimensional Diagnosis of Personality – Not Whether but When and Which'. The DSM-5 Personality Disorders Work Group laboured long and hard to develop its own dimensional system, but it was finally rejected as too unreliable, untested, and impossibly complicated for routine clinical practice.

The ICD-11 has eliminated the diagnosis of the separate personality disorders altogether. Instead, the clinician need decide only if personality disorder is present or absent; if present, whether it is mild, moderate, or severe; and whether it features negative affectivity, detachment, anankastia, dissociality, and disinhibition. Unfortunately, this new ICD-11 system is inherently unreliable and unworkable. If it's hard enough to operationally define the individual personality disorders and achieve rater agreement on their presence or absence, it seems impossible to get agreement on the presence or absence of the much more abstract construct of Personality Disorder. The ICD-11 approach is entirely new, disturbingly radical, completely unfamiliar, and totally untested. It was developed by a small group of enthusiastic experts, without much input from the field, without a compelling literature review, and without extensive field testing in a variety of clinical and cultural settings. The ICD-11 system of Personality Disorder is well meaning, but half-baked and not ready for prime time. I doubt it will be much used or serve much purpose. (Editor's note: it should be noted that all published clinical comparisons of ICD-11 and ICD-10 personality disorder (now seven) have concluded that ICD-11 is superior to ICD-10, but in stating this the Editor has to acknowledge he was Chair of the ICD-11 Revision Group for Personality Disorder so bias may not be far away. But none of these comparisons have involved him.)

Disorders New to ICD-11 That Were Included in DSM-IV or DSM-5

Bipolar II Disorder

On balance, I regret adding Bipolar II to DSM-IV and worry it may be similarly misused by clinicians using ICD-11. Identifying Bipolar II is valuable because it may help reduce iatrogenic switches to mania and rapid cycling in Bipolar spectrum patients receiving antidepressants without the coverage of mood stabilizers. Patients with a Bipolar II pattern of symptoms also sort with Bipolar Disorder in family history, course, treatment response, and outcome. Unfortunately, these advantages are offset by the great disadvantage that

Bipolar II became a fad diagnosis promoted by drug companies – leading to much iatrogenic harm caused by massive overuse of antipsychotic drugs. Bipolar II is an excellent diagnosis when used carefully, but does more iatrogenic harm than good when used carelessly.

Catatonia

Making Catatonia a separate new category in ICD-11 is among the few of its decisions I heartily and unreservedly endorse. For too long, clinicians have assumed that catatonic symptoms have some special relationship to Schizophrenia. As a result of mislabelling, the real cause of the catatonic symptoms was often missed; the proper treatment not given; the patient stigmatized with an inaccurate schizophrenia label and subjected to the overuse of antipsychotic medications. Catatonic symptoms are in fact more usually caused by neurological illness; bipolar disorder; or substance use – and the causal disorder should be the focus of treatment. Missing an underlying medical cause of Catatonia can be catastrophic. Benzodiazepines or electroconvulsive therapy are specific and quickly effective in the emergency situations that sometimes accompany Catatonia, antipsychotics much less so.

Binge Eating Disorder (BED)

The first suggestion to make Binge Eating Disorder (BED) an official diagnosis was offered by the eating disorder experts working on DSM-IV. They reported seeing patients who needed help for binge eating, but who didn't fulfil the full criteria for Bulimia Nervosa (BN). Bulimia Nervosa required that the patient's binges be compensated via dieting, vomiting, laxatives, or intense exercise. BED would be for those who binged without any of these compensatory behaviours – and who were therefore more likely to become overweight or obese. We had a high threshold for including new disorders in DSM-IV and BED didn't come close to making the cut. The DSM-5 radically lowered the bar for including new diagnoses, giving its experts free rein to promote their pets. The few, largely uninformative studies supporting BED were enough to achieve DSM-5 approval – and now ICD-11 has followed suit. Why does this worry me? A drug company received expedited US Food and Drug Administration approval to peddle its ADHD pill (relabelled 'Vyvance') for BED. This was based on only a few, small, inadequate, short-term treatment trials that had failed to demonstrate any compelling, clinically significant, enduring benefit. Because the FDA is heavily funded by the drug industry that it is supposed to regulate, it now seems to work much more for the corporations than for the public. The drug company spared no expense pushing its stimulant drug, hiring a former world tennis champ to appear in its ads. The result is that annual sales are now close to $3 billion, despite the fact there is no convincing evidence that diet pills have any long-lasting impact on either binging behaviour or weight gain. Because binge eating is such a ubiquitous symptom among normals, the ICD-11 decision to include Binge Eating Disorder is likely to cause massive overdiagnosis and diet pill popping.

Premenstrual Dysphoric Disorder

Whether or not to include Premenstrual Dysphoric Disorder was the most controversial decision facing DSM-IV. We deferred it pending additional research – and the diagnosis was subsequently accepted by both DSM-5 and ICD-11. There were strong arguments both ways. Some women have 'severe mood, somatic, or cognitive symptoms that begin several days before the onset of menses, start to improve within a few days, and become minimal or absent within a week'. To make the diagnosis, this must be a recurring and enduring pattern that causes clinically significant distress or impairment. The strong opposition to including Premenstrual Dysphoric Disorder was based on the reasonable fear that it would be misused to overdiagnose, overtreat, objectify, pathologize, and stigmatize normal bodily changes in women. On balance, this is a useful diagnosis – but only if used cautiously in clear-cut cases.

'Hoarding Disorder'

'Hoarding Disorder' was introduced by DSM-5 under pressure from a small group of researchers who believe it to be a sufficiently distinct set of behaviours to merit its own category. The ICD-11 has followed suit. There are two problems not given sufficient weight in making this decision. First, hoarding is an associated feature of many psychiatric disorders including Schizophrenia; OCD; Mood Disorders; Autism; and Dementia – and also of some neurological disorders. Hoarding is also a widespread normal behaviour, especially common as people age, accumulate more goods, become more nostalgic. 'Hoarding Disorder' can be a useful diagnosis if restricted to the very small group of patients who have it as a primary symptom at a degree of severity that causes serious harms, risks, or malfunctions. It is a harmful diagnosis if, on the severe end, it distracts from a careful differential diagnosis of underlying causes or, on the mild end, pathologizes normal behaviour.

Conclusions

The best way to use ICD-11 is with extreme caution. All of its new diagnoses are on the heavily populated, very fuzzy border with normality. Patients presenting with severe mental disorders can usually be diagnosed reliably and with confidence. In contrast, patients presenting with milder problems, particularly of the sort included in the untested new diagnoses introduced by ICD-11, would probably most often be better off if not diagnosed at all. Many people have the symptoms described as ICD-11 essential features, without having the clinically significant level of distress and impairment that must be present before diagnosing a mental disorder. Underdiagnosis of mild problems is almost always less risky and more accurate than overdiagnosis. Underdiagnoses can be corrected; overdiagnosis often leads irrevocably to unnecessary stigma and overmedication. Diagnoses are easy to make, but extremely hard ever to erase. I have seen many patients haunted for life by a misdiagnosis that was made carelessly in just 10 minutes.

Patients would probably be better off if psychiatric diagnosis had been frozen 50 years ago with the publication of DSM-III – before the accretion of so many questionable new disorders and the massive overdiagnosis and overtreatment that have since followed. The pace of growth of scientific understanding has been ever so much slower than the pace of diagnostic exuberance and inflation. The American Psychiatric Association did terribly poorly in generating DSM-5 and this has generally proven itself a poor custodian of psychiatric diagnosis. The APA has abundant resources to devote to the task of DSM production, but is wasteful in using them and influenced by its glaring financial conflict of interest – the huge profits it makes as publisher of the DSM franchise encourages it to favour novelty. The World Health Organization also did an awful job on ICD-11 in large part for the opposite reason – it had a tiny budget and was almost totally dependent on volunteer experts who were allowed to run wild with their pet suggestions for untried new diagnoses.

Antipsychiatry types exploit the obvious flaws and limitations of both DSM-5 and ICD-11 to promote the idea that all psychiatric diagnosis is unnecessary. I could not disagree more. I don't trust clinicians who know only psychiatric diagnosis, but I equally distrust those who know it not at all and criticize it out of ignorance or sectarian interest. Psychiatric diagnosis is never sufficient for creating accurate formulations and choosing best treatment plans – but it is always necessary. Clinicians unskilled in psychiatric diagnosis do a grave disservice to their patients.

Having two flawed/risky systems of psychiatric diagnosis is much worse than having just one – but expecting a future union of ICD and DSM into one good/safe system would be a naive triumph of hope over experience. The APA will hang on to its DSM cash cow with ferocious greed and WHO will never have sufficient budget to control the diagnostic exuberance of its advisors. And there is no other agency waiting in the wings, willing and able to do a better job. People around the world accustomed to using DSM will continue to use its future editions. People around the world accustomed to ICD will stick with it. The best we can probably hope for is educating clinicians to do their best to avoid overdiagnosis and overtreatment, whichever of the two overinclusive systems they are using. That cautioning of clinicians has been my purpose here..

Editor's note: Allen Frances' writings are always a sparkling and enjoyable read, but while many people would be warmed by attendance at the bonfire of both of the diagnostic systems he describes, I encourage the reader to read the rest of the book when they are ready to cool down. Then they can come to a final opinion.

Chapter 3
Schizophrenia or Other Primary Psychotic Disorders

Wolfgang Gaebel & Eva Salveridou-Hof

Introduction

The term 'psychosis' was originally introduced in 1845 by Ernst Freiherr von Feuchtersleben, a poet and medical doctor, and was used later to describe severe mental disorders. Nowadays, psychosis denotes a clinical syndrome, not a nosological entity, which is characterized by significant impairments and alterations in experience and behaviour usually manifest in positive symptoms such as persistent delusions, persistent hallucinations, disorganized thinking (typically disorganized speech), grossly disorganized behaviour, experiences of passivity and control, negative symptoms such as blunted or flat affect and avolition, and psychomotor disturbances.

A psychotic syndrome may be due to primary psychiatric disorders such as schizophrenia or to secondary psychiatric disorders such as substance use or medical conditions coded elsewhere in ICD-11. Psychotic symptoms should occur with sufficient frequency and intensity to deviate from expected cultural or subcultural norms. They do not arise as a feature of another mental and behavioural disorder (e.g., a mood disorder, delirium, or a disorder due to substance use).

To the best of present knowledge, psychotic disorders have variable phenotypic expressions and are still poorly understood despite an enormous amount of research findings.[1,2] They comprise a complex a etiopathogenesis, involving a major genetic contribution, as well as environmental factors interacting with genetic susceptibility, but cannot yet be defined or diagnosed by laboratory tests or genetic or neuroimaging techniques.

Origins of the Concept of Schizophrenia

The most common psychotic disorder is schizophrenia. Emil Kraepelin (1856–1926) proposed to integrate mental disease entities based on the overall clinical picture of symptoms, course, and outcome into a single nosological entity under the name of 'dementia praecox'. It was based on his longitudinal observations of a large number of clinical cases exhibiting a common pattern resulting in poor prognosis with severe cognitive and social decline.[3,4]

Eugen Bleuler (1857–1939) significantly modified Kraepelin's original concept. In 1911, he coined the name 'schizophrenia' (from the Greek *schizein* (splitting) and *phren* (soul, spirit, mind)), giving his monograph the title 'Dementia Praecox or the Group of Schizophrenias', subscribing in his opinion to the separation of different types of schizophrenia with putatively different aetiologies, psychopathology, course, and outcome – and therefore prognosis.

Importantly, Bleuler introduced a distinction between fundamental (obligatory) and accessory (supplementary) symptoms of the disorder.[5] While the accessory symptoms comprised hallucinations and delusions, which could wax and wane over the course of illness, the fundamental symptoms included thought and speech derailment, such as loss of associations, inappropriate affect, ambivalence, avolition, and autism, which he described as existing throughout the illness course. Additionally, he described primary and secondary symptoms, the former indicating closer connection to the biological substrate of the disorder.

During the ensuing decades, further subcategories within the broadening phenotype of schizophrenia were described.[6] Later, Kurt Schneider (1887–1967) designated psychotic manifestations as 'first-rank symptoms', such as hearing commenting or conversing voices, thoughts being inserted or withdrawn, other feelings of alien influence, and other ego-disturbances as having a decisive weight in the diagnosis of schizophrenia, although not being pathognomonic.[7]

Nowadays, psychotic disorders are divided into primary and secondary disorders. Whereas primary psychosis is a psychiatric disorder *sui generis* of still unknown a etiopathogenesis, secondary psychosis may be caused by specific medical conditions. Although patients with primary psychosis are likely to have auditory hallucinations, prominent cognitive disorders, and complex delusions, those with secondary psychosis may exhibit cognitive changes, abnormal vital signs, and visual hallucinations. However, differential diagnosis by the nature of psychopathology alone usually does not allow clear separation without the additional use of neuropsychiatric and/or additional specialized medical assessment.

The new ICD-11 category 'Schizophrenia or Other Primary Psychotic Disorders' is part of the ICD-11 Chapter 6, 'Mental, Behavioural or Neurodevelopmental Disorder'. These disorders are described as 'syndromes characterised by clinically significant disturbance in an individual's cognition, emotional regulation, or behaviour that reflects a dysfunction in the psychological, biological, or developmental processes that underlie mental and behavioural functioning. These disturbances are usually associated with distress or impairment in personal, family, social, educational, occupational, or other important areas of functioning' (icd.who.int).

Changes from ICD-10 to ICD-11: What Is New?

The ICD-11 grouping of schizophrenia or other primary psychotic disorders replaces the ICD-10 F2 grouping of schizophrenia, schizotypal, and delusional disorders. ICD-11 describes this group as follows (icd.who.int., 2021):

> Schizophrenia or other primary psychotic disorders are characterised by significant impairments in reality testing and alterations in behaviour manifest in positive symptoms such as persistent delusions, persistent hallucinations, disorganised thinking (typically manifest as disorganised speech), grossly disorganised behaviour, and experiences of passivity and control, negative symptoms such as blunted or flat affect and avolition, and psychomotor disturbances. The symptoms occur with sufficient frequency and intensity to deviate from expected cultural or subcultural norms. These symptoms do not arise as a feature of another mental and behavioural disorder (e.g., a mood disorder, delirium, or a disorder due to substance use). The categories in this grouping should not be used to classify the expression of ideas, beliefs, or behaviours that are culturally sanctioned.

one's feelings, impulses, thoughts, or behaviour are under the control of an external force), cognition (e.g., impaired attention, verbal memory, and social cognition), volition (e.g., loss of motivation), affect (e.g., blunted emotional expression), and behaviour (e.g., behaviour that appears bizarre or purposeless, unpredictable or inappropriate emotional responses that interfere with the organisation of behaviour). Psychomotor disturbances, including catatonia, may be present. Persistent delusions, persistent hallucinations, thought disorder, and experiences of influence, passivity, or control are considered core symptoms. Symptoms must have persisted for at least one month in order for a diagnosis of schizophrenia to be assigned. The symptoms are not a manifestation of another health condition (e.g., a brain tumour) and are not due to the effect of a substance or medication on the central nervous system (e.g., corticosteroids), including withdrawal (e.g., alcohol withdrawal)' (icd.who.int).

The diagnosis requires at least two of seven symptom categories, of which one symptom must be from group a) through d) that are present most of the time for a period of 1 month or more.

Symptoms include:

a) Persistent delusions (e.g., grandiose delusions, delusions of reference, persecutory delusions),
b) Persistent hallucinations (most commonly auditory, although they may be in any sensory modality),
c) Disorganized thinking (formal thought disorder, e.g., tangential and loose associations, irrelevant speech, neologisms),
d) Experiences of influence, passivity, or control (i.e., the experience that one's feelings, impulses, actions, or thoughts are not generated by oneself, are being placed in one's mind or withdrawn from one's mind by others, or that one's thoughts are being broadcast to others),
e) Negative symptoms such as affective flattening, alogia, or paucity of speech, avolition, asociality, and anhedonia,
f) Grossly disorganized behaviour that impedes goal-directed activity (e.g., behaviour that appears bizarre or purposeless, unpredictable or inappropriate emotional responses that interfere with the ability to organize behaviour),
g) Psychomotor disturbances such as catatonic restlessness or agitation, posturing, waxy flexibility, negativism, mutism, or stupor.

The symptoms are not manifestations of another medical condition (e.g., a brain tumour) and are not due to the effects of a substance or medication (e.g., corticosteroids) on the central nervous system, including withdrawal effects (e.g., from alcohol).

Schizophrenia is frequently associated with significant distress and significant impairment in personal, family, social, educational, occupational, or other important areas of functioning. However, distress and psychosocial impairment are not requirements for a diagnosis of schizophrenia.

Additional features include that the onset of schizophrenia might be acute, with serious disturbance apparent within a few days, or with a gradual development of signs and symptoms. A prodromal phase often precedes the onset of psychotic symptoms by weeks or months. The characteristic features of this phase often include loss of interest in work or social activities, neglect of personal appearance or hygiene, inversion of the sleep cycle, and attenuated psychotic symptoms, accompanied by negative symptoms, anxiety/agitation, or varying degrees of depressive symptoms. Between acute episodes there may be residual phases, which are similar phenomenologically to the prodromal phase.

The course of schizophrenia is variable. Some patients experience exacerbations and remission of symptoms periodically throughout their lives, others a gradual worsening of symptoms, and a smaller proportion experience complete remission of symptoms. Positive symptoms tend to diminish naturally over time, whereas negative symptoms often persist and are closely tied to poorer prognosis. Cognitive symptoms also tend to be more persistent and when present are associated with ongoing functional impairment.

Although schizophrenia can occur at any age, the average age of onset tends to be in the late teens to the early 20s for men, and the late 20s to early 30s for women. Cultural factors may influence the onset, symptom pattern, course, and outcome of schizophrenia. Among migrants and ethnic and cultural minorities, living in areas with a low proportion of their own ethnic, migrant, or cultural group, there are higher rates of schizophrenia. As a whole, it is more prevalent among males.[14,15]

'Schizoaffective disorder is an episodic disorder in which the diagnostic requirements of schizophrenia and a manic, mixed, or moderate or severe depressive episode are met within the same episode of illness, either simultaneously or within a few days of each other. Prominent symptoms of schizophrenia (e.g., delusions, hallucinations, characterised in the form of thought, experiences of influence, passivity and control) are accompanied by typical symptoms of a moderate or severe depressive episode (e.g., depressed mood, loss of interest, reduced energy), a manic episode (e.g., an extreme mood state characterized by euphoria, irritability, or expansiveness; increased activity or a subjective experience of increased energy) or a mixed episode. Psychomotor disturbances, including catatonia, may be present. Symptoms must have persisted for at least one month. The symptoms are not a manifestation of another medical condition (e.g., a brain tumour) and are not due to the effect of a substance or medication on the central nervous system (e.g., corticosteroids), including withdrawal (e.g., alcohol withdrawal)'.[14]

Additional clinical features describe that the onset of schizoaffective disorder may be acute, with serious disturbance apparent within a few days, or with gradual development of signs and symptoms. There is often a history of prior mood episodes and a previous diagnosis of a depressive disorder or a bipolar disorder.[15]

'Schizotypal disorder is characterised by an enduring pattern (i.e., characteristic of the person's functioning over a period of at least several years) of eccentricities in behaviour, appearance and speech, accompanied by cognitive and perceptual distortions, unusual beliefs, and discomfort with – and often reduced capacity for – interpersonal relationships. Symptoms may include constricted or inappropriate affect and anhedonia. Paranoid ideas, ideas of reference, or other psychotic symptoms, including hallucinations in any modality, may occur, but are not of sufficient intensity or duration to meet the diagnostic requirements of schizophrenia, schizoaffective disorder, or delusional disorder. The symptoms cause distress or impairment in personal, family, social, educational, occupational or other important areas of functioning'.[14]

Schizotypal disorder is more common in biological relatives of persons with a diagnosis of schizophrenia and is considered to be part of the spectrum of schizophrenia-related psychopathology. It begins in late adolescence or early adulthood, without a definite age of onset.[15]

'Acute and transient psychotic disorder (ATPD) is characterised by acute onset of psychotic symptoms that emerge without a prodrome and reach their maximal severity within two weeks. Symptoms may include delusions, hallucinations, disorganisation of thought processes, perplexity or confusion, and disturbances of affect and mood. Catatonia-like psychomotor disturbances may be present. Symptoms typically change rapidly, both in nature and intensity, from day to day, or even within a single day. The duration of the episode does not exceed 3 months, and most commonly lasts from a few days to 1 month. The symptoms are not a manifestation of another medical condition (e.g., a brain tumour) and are not due to the effect of a substance or medication on the central nervous system (e.g., corticosteroids), including withdrawal (e.g., alcohol withdrawal)'.[14]

The onset of ATPD is usually associated with rapid deterioration in social and occupational functioning. The disorder may occur during adolescence or later in the lifespan often following an episode of acute stress.[15]

'Delusional disorder is characterised by the development of a delusion or set of related delusions, typically persisting for at least 3 months and often much longer, in the absence of a Depressive, Manic, or Mixed mood episode. The delusions are variable in content across individuals, but typically stable within individuals, although they may evolve over time. Other characteristic symptoms of Schizophrenia (i.e., clear and persistent hallucinations, negative symptoms, disorganised thinking, or experiences of influence, passivity, or control) are not present, although various forms of perceptual disturbances (e.g., hallucinations, illusions, misidentifications of persons) thematically related to the delusion are still consistent with the diagnosis. Apart from actions and attitudes directly related to the delusion or delusional system, affect, speech, and behavior are typically unaffected. The symptoms are not a manifestation of another medical condition (e.g., a brain tumour) and are not due to the effect of a substance or medication on the central nervous system (e.g., corticosteroids), including withdrawal effects (e.g., alcohol withdrawal)'.[14]

Delusional disorder typically has a later onset and greater stability of symptoms than other psychotic disorders with delusional symptoms.[15]

Diagnostic Boundaries and Differential Diagnosis

Boundaries with normality: Psychotic experiences may occur in the general population, but do not last long enough to qualify for a disorder and/or are not accompanied by functional impairment. In schizophrenia, multiple persistent symptoms are present and are often accompanied by impairment in cognitive functioning and other psychosocial fields. Cultural variations in experience may appear psychotic, but it should be determined whether the experience is normative or accepted within the culture before assigning a diagnosis.

Boundaries with mood disorders: Psychotic symptoms may occur during moderate or severe depressive, manic, or mixed episodes, often with content consistent with mood state. However, they occur only during the mood episode, and do not meet the duration requirement for schizophrenia so as to qualify for schizoaffective disorder.

Distinguishing between Schizophrenia and Schizoaffective Disorder

In both disorders, at least two characteristic symptoms are present most of the time for a period of 1 month or more. In schizoaffective disorder, the symptoms of schizophrenia are present concurrently with mood symptoms that meet the full diagnostic requirements of a mood episode and last for at least 1 month. In contrast, in schizophrenia co-occurring mood symptoms, if any, either do not persist for as long as 1 month or are not of sufficient severity to meet the requirements of a moderate or severe depressive episode, a manic episode, or a mixed episode.

Distinguishing between Schizophrenia and Acute and Transient Psychotic Disorder

The psychotic symptoms of schizophrenia persist for at least 1 month in their full, florid form. In contrast, the symptoms of ATPD tend to fluctuate rapidly in intensity and type across time. Further negative symptoms present in schizophrenia do not occur in ATPD.

Distinguishing between Schizophrenia and Schizotypal Disorder

Schizophrenia is differentiated from schizotypal disorder entirely on the intensity of the symptoms. Schizophrenia is diagnosed if the symptoms are sufficiently intense to meet its diagnostic requirements.

Distinguishing between Schizophrenia and Delusional Disorder

Both schizophrenia and delusional disorder may be characterized by persistent delusions. If other features are present that meet the diagnostic requirements of schizophrenia, a diagnosis of schizophrenia should be made. However, hallucinations that are consistent with the content of the delusions and do not occur persistently are consistent with a diagnosis of delusional disorder.[15]

Common Comorbidities

Schizophrenia most often remains a disorder with a relapsing or chronic course, cognitive and functional impairment, and a reduced life expectancy (between 15 and 25 years). Its management can be challenging, particularly in the presence of comorbid conditions that can affect the clinical course, treatment response, and outcome.[16,17] Some comorbid disorders may precede the onset of schizophrenia, whereas others emerge or become clinically prominent after its onset.[18]

People with schizophrenia have a statistically significant higher risk for metabolic and cardiovascular diseases, cancer, pulmonary disease, and other medical comorbidities.[19,20]

In particular, psychiatric comorbidities, such as depression, obsessive–compulsive disorder, or substance abuse, are common among patients with schizophrenia and are recognized as an important clinical problem in diagnosis, treatment, and care.

Conversely, some neurological comorbidities, such as movement disorders (e.g., Parkinson's disease), may play a role in the pathophysiology of schizophrenia, and some somatic comorbidities, such as diabetes and obesity, may be secondary to the pharmacotherapy and unhealthy lifestyle associated with schizophrenia. Substance use comorbidities (e.g., alcohol, cannabis, stimulants) may play a role in triggering the onset of schizophrenia or contribute to medical comorbidities (e.g., liver disease, HIV). Suicide is the largest, although not the only, contributor to the decreased life expectancy in individuals with schizophrenia.[21]

Independent of the illness phase, in addition to guideline-based pharmacotherapy, psychotherapy, and psychosocial therapy it is recommended to offer people with schizophrenia regular monitoring of their physical health, especially in people with schizophrenia and high blood pressure, abnormal lipid levels, obesity and/or diabetes, and those who smoke or who are not physically active.[22]

Comparison with DSM-5 Equivalent Diagnoses

The ICD-11 classification of mental disorders and the DSM-5 were developed during overlapping time periods. Thereby, the organization of the diagnostic groupings in the metastructure of both systems was partly harmonized.

Nevertheless, there are significant differences between the classification systems beginning with the naming of the psychotic disorder groups. In ICD-11, the category is named 'Schizophrenia or other primary psychotic disorders', while in DSM-5 the category is named 'Schizophrenia Spectrum and other psychotic disorders'.

Furthermore, the ICD-11 and DSM-5 diagnostic requirements for schizophrenia differ in several ways:[23]

- The required minimum duration for schizophrenia in ICD-11 definition is 'a period of 1 month or more', whereas DSM-5 requires that 'continuous signs of the disturbance persist for at least 6 months'. The DSM-5 requirement for an additional 5 months of symptoms can include prodromal or residual symptoms. Although both diagnostic systems require a full month of the defining psychotic symptoms, the DSM-5 diagnostic requirements are more likely to identify patients with a higher tendency to chronicity.[24]
- ICD-11's shorter duration requirement, along with the introduction of a first-episode course qualifier, is intended to encourage earlier initiation of appropriate treatment, which has been shown to improve patient outcomes.[25]
- The required pattern of symptoms of schizophrenia differs as well. While both DSM-5 and ICD-11 require at least two types of symptoms lasting at least 1 month, ICD-11 includes 'experiences of influence, passivity or control' as a separate core symptom. These disturbances in the 'ego–world boundary' involve patients having experiences such as their thoughts, actions, or emotions being imposed by an outside force (passivity experiences), their thoughts being physically removed from their mind (thought withdrawal), or their thoughts being transmitted to others (thought broadcasting). Such disturbances were included among Schneider's first-rank symptoms, which he considered to be characteristic of schizophrenia in the absence of organic conditions.[7] Although first-rank symptoms have been de-emphasized in ICD-11,[10] experiences of influence, passivity, or control were judged to be sufficiently important and distinctive to be retained. In DSM-5, these symptoms are examples of delusions, while ICD-11 keeps 'experiences' separate from the delusions ('beliefs').
- While DSM-5 restricts negative symptoms of schizophrenia to diminished emotional expression and avolition, ICD-11 also includes alogia or paucity of speech, asociality, and anhedonia. Furthermore, DSM-5 requires a deterioration in functioning in one or more major areas, such as work, interpersonal relations, or self-care, since the onset of the disturbance. There is no such requirement in ICD-11, although the text mentions that the diagnosis is 'frequently associated' with significant functional impairment.

- Although DSM-5 and ICD-11 both allow specification of the level of severity for various symptom domains, these domains and their assessment are somewhat different in the two systems. While ICD-11 identifies six symptom domains rated on a 4-point scale (not present, mild, moderate, severe) DSM-5 identifies three separate domains (hallucinations, delusions, disorganized speech) corresponding to the single ICD-11 positive symptom dimension, in addition to the domains of negative symptoms, impaired cognition, abnormal psychomotor behaviour, depression, and mania. These domains are rated on a 5-point scale (not present, equivocal, mild, moderate, severe). In the DSM-5, these ratings are included in Section III, 'Emerging Measures and Models', and not in Section II, 'Diagnostic Criteria and Codes', whereas in the ICD-11 they appear in the main body of the Clinical Descriptions and Diagnostic Requirements (CDDR).
- The DSM-5 category of schizophreniform disorder, which differs from schizophrenia primarily with respect to the duration of symptoms, is not included in ICD-11 but would correspond to one of the residual categories 6A2Y or 6A2Z.

Moreover, there are differences between ICD-11 and DSM-5 in their conceptualization of schizoaffective disorder (SAD). In ICD-11, the diagnostic requirements for schizophrenia have to be met concurrently with those for a moderate or severe depressive episode, a manic episode, or a mixed episode, with a duration of at least 1 month, and an onset of the psychotic and mood symptoms either simultaneously or within a few days of each other. Because this definition focuses on the pattern of symptoms during the current episode, an individual's presentation can meet the diagnostic requirements for schizoaffective disorder, schizophrenia, or a mood disorder during different episodes of their illness.

In contrast, the DSM-5 diagnostic criteria in a longitudinal concept of SAD involve a retrospective assessment of the interplay between mood and psychotic symptoms across the entire course of the disturbance. The DSM-5 requires that there be: a) an uninterrupted period of illness during which there is a major depressive or manic episode concurrent with the symptomatic criteria for schizophrenia; b) a period of delusions or hallucinations lasting at least 2 weeks occurring in the absence of a major depressive or manic episode at some point during the lifetime duration of the illness; and c) symptoms that meet criteria for a major depressive or manic episode for the majority of the total duration of the active and residual portions of the illness.

Whereas DSM-5 categorizes a 'sequential' symptom type of SAD, ICD-11 describes (as does ICD-10, but with less stringent criteria) a 'concurrent' symptom type.[26] From both types, resulting 'polymorphous' course types (various types of episodes over time) are much more frequent (70%) than 'monomorphous' ones (same type of episodes over time). Hence, changing episodes over time in SAD are more the rule than the exception, independent of the classification system. DSM-5, relying for the diagnosis on the retrospective assessment of the interplay of psychotic and mood symptoms, is more at risk for reliability problems.[23]

The ICD-11 category of Acute and transient psychotic disorder involves the acute onset of psychotic symptoms within 2 weeks, changing rapidly both in nature and intensity from day to day, and lasting up to 3 months. The closest available DSM-5 category, Brief psychotic disorder, is based entirely on the duration of psychotic symptoms (less than 1 month) and has no requirement for fluctuating symptomatology.

Advantages of the ICD-11 Classification of Mental, Behavioural, or Neurodevelopmental Disorders (MBND)

Overall, the coding system in the newest revision of the International Classification of Diseases and Related Health Problems (ICD-11) is more contemporary and user-friendly and is offering resources such as the online Coding Tool, Implementation or Transition Guide, and Reference Guide. It has provided major changes to bring the ICD classification of mental and behavioural disorders in line with current empirical evidence and clinical practice.

Field studies that assess how well the proposed changes perform were conducted in a broad spectrum of mental health care settings across countries with varied languages, cultures, and resource levels.[27] The results of these studies show that all common and high-burden disorders in the adult population were diagnosed with at least satisfactory and in most cases excellent reliabilities, suggesting that the proposed ICD-11 is suitable for use and commonly applicable at a global level.

The ICD-11 disorders are presented in terms of the essential features that clinicians could reasonably expect to find in all cases, in an effort to communicate the essence of the disorder, with greater flexibility for clinicians and cultural variation.

In general, the reliability of diagnoses in ICD-11 was superior to that of diagnoses in ICD-10, though strict comparisons are not appropriate due to differences in methodology of these field studies. Reliability coefficients were based on routine clinical assessments using open form interviews by clinicians with diverse training and experience. The results were similar to those achieved by diagnostic assessments using more complex and time-consuming instruments. These observations suggest that the use of more uniform procedures by clinicians based on a brief training may yield adequate reliability for commonly diagnosed mental disorders in clinical settings.[28]

In addition, a set of dimensional qualifiers has also been introduced to describe the symptomatic manifestations of schizophrenia or other primary psychotic disorders, giving the possibility of a stronger person-specific categorical diagnostic and therapy indication.[10] Rather than focusing on diagnostic subtypes, the dimensional approach to classification focuses on relevant aspects of the current clinical presentation in ways that are much more consistent with recovery-based psychiatric rehabilitation approaches. For the ICD-11 CDDR, working groups were asked to deliver their recommendations as 'content forms', including consistent and systematic information for each disorder that provided the basis for the diagnostic guidelines.

An international web-based study provided insights into how well the ICD-11 functions when applied by health professionals. Overall, the use led to an increased percentage of correctly selected diagnoses compared with ICD-10. Additionally, participants' experiences with ICD-11 were rated as remarkably positive. The time required for making a diagnosis was lower and ratings of clinical utility more favourable for ICD-11 compared with ICD-10, improvements having been shown for judgements on the ease of use and related utility measures. Whereas diagnostic consistency on average was better for ICD-11 compared with ICD-10 based on the use of diagnostic guidelines for case vignettes by mental health professionals, coding consistency based on coding instructions and brief diagnostic descriptions by the same participants was slightly poorer in ICD-11 compared with ICD-10, underscoring the need of more intense training.[29,30]

Symptom and course qualifiers are allowing to diagnose and code more personalized symptom- and course-profiles over time and thus to make more individualized judgements for treatment and care with presumably better outcomes, which remains to be investigated by further field studies. Taken together, these findings should be interpreted as indicators for a positive outcome of the ICD-revision process and its advantages in general.

Discussion

The development of the ICD-11 for Mental, Behavioural, or Neurodevelopmental Disorders and their underlying statistical classification represents the first major revision of the world's foremost classification of mental disorders in nearly 30 years. In the development of the ICD-11 MBND chapter, substantial changes have been made to ensure clinical utility, global applicability, and scientific validity in the light of current evidence. There were also notable steps towards dimensionality regarding symptom severity and time course.

An initial goal of the ICD-11 CDDG development process was to create a mechanism to ensure consistent and relatively uniform provision of diagnostic information across the various categories. Therefore, the availability of the digital ICD-11 maintenance and proposal platform to upload empirically based relevant commentaries or proposals allows a steady improvement of the diagnostic classification. Further, the implementation of a new classification system involves the interaction of the classification with each country's laws, policies, health systems, and information infrastructure. Multiple modalities must be developed for training a broad range of international health professionals.

The ICD-11 diagnostic guidelines for use in clinical settings have undergone rigorous field testing – changes in the diagnostic guidelines from ICD-10 to ICD-11 are reflecting the outcome of ongoing developments in nosological science. These modifications, together with the option for digitally supported complex coding embedded in a 'content model' with its diagnostic core of 'essential features' and the other domains, allow for a composite categorical and dimensional diagnostic classification with a longitudinal and cross-sectional type of course staging and symptom profiling. Thereby, clinicians are enabled to select a more person-oriented treatment and care.[31]

On the basis of these developments, the modified schizophrenia construct is still alive and viable and will most probably even improve contemporary clinical practice globally.[30]

In conclusion, the new mental disorders classification in ICD-11 and its accompanying diagnostic guidelines represent an important advance for the field. The revised schizophrenia category from the perspectives of applicability, utility, and reliability has salvaged the construct for clinical practice until new approaches demonstrate superiority in validity (and utility) – and in stimulating the development of superior versions of treatment and care in correspondingly adapted mental health care systems. This, however, would take time to manage transition, implementation, and adaptation of a new construct (including education and training for the mental health workforce). Instead, for example, a pilot model of a deconstructed schizophrenia version would need to be evaluated as well as, and in comparison with, the current classification version. Validating such a partly new if not supplanting construct would, of course, need adequate scientific strategies and methodologies depending on the kind of innovation. All of this would take several years, during which the diagnostics, treatment, and care according to the ICD-11 construct would remain in place.[32]

References

1. Vyas, N.S., Patel, N.H., Puri, B.K. (2011). Neurobiology and phenotypic expression in early onset schizophrenia. *Early Interv Psychiatry*, **5**(1), 3–14. https://doi.org/10.1111/j.1751-7893.2010.00253.x

2. van Os, J., Linscott, R.J. (2012). Introduction: the extended psychosis phenotype-relationship with schizophrenia and with ultrahigh risk status for psychosis. *Schizophr Bull*, **38**(2), 227–230. https://doi.org/10.1093/schbul/sbr188

3. Kraepelin, E. (1899). *Psychiatrie*. 6 Auflage. Leipzig, Austria: Barth. English translation by Metoui, H., Ayed, S. (1990). *Psychiatry, A Textbook for Students and Physicians*. Canton, MA: Science History Publications.

4. Kraepelin, E. (1909). *Psychiatrie*. 8 Auflage. Leipzig, Austria: Barth. English translation and adaptation by Barclay, R.M., Robertson, G.M. (1919). *Dementia Praecox and Paraphrenia*. Huntington, NY: Krieger Publishing. Reprinted 1971.

5. Bleuler, E. (1911). *Dementia praecox oder Gruppe der Schizophrenien*. Berlin, Leipzig and Vienna: F. Deuticke.

6. Jablensky, A. (2011). Diagnosis and revision of the classification systems. In Gaebel, W. (Ed.), *Schizophrenia: Current Science and Clinical Practice*, pp. 1–30. Wiley-Blackwell. https://doi.org/10.1002/9780470978672.ch1

7. Schneider, K. (1950). *Klinische Psychopathologie*. Stuttgart, Germany: Thieme. English translation by Hamilton, M.W., Anderson, E.W. (1959). *Clinical Psychopathology*, 8th ed. New York: Grune and Stratton.

8. Nordgaard, J., Arnfred, S.M., Handest, P., Parnas, J. (2008). The diagnostic status of first-rank symptoms. *Schizophr Bull*, **34**, 137–154.

9. Tandon, R., Nasrallah, H. A., Keshavan, M. S. (2009). Schizophrenia, 'just the facts' 4. Clinical features and conceptualization. *Schizophr Res*, **110**(1-3), 1–23. https://doi.org/10.1016/j.schres.2009.03.005

10. Gaebel, W. (2012). Status of psychotic disorders in ICD-11. *Schizophr Bull*, **38**(5), 895–898.

11. Bromet, E.J., Naz, B., Fochtmann, L.J., Carlson, G.A., Tanenberg-Karant, M. (2005). Long-term diagnostic stability and outcome in recent first-episode cohort studies of schizophrenia. *Schizophr Bull*, **31**, 639–649.

12. Green, M.F., Kern, R.S., Heaton, R.K. (2004).). Longitudinal studies of cognition and functional outcome in schizophrenia: implications for MATRICS. *Schizophr Res*. **72**, 41–51.

13. Reed, G.M., First, M.B., Kogan, C.S., et al. (2019). Innovations and changes in the ICD-11 classification of mental, behavioural and neurodevelopmental disorders. *World Psychiatry*, **18**(1), 3–19. https://doi.org/10.1002/wps.20611

14. World Health Organization. (2021). *International Classification of Diseases 11th Revision*. (icd.who.int)

15. Global Clinical Practice Network. (2021). (gcp.network)

16. Kilbourne, A.M., Morden, N.E., Austin, K., et al. (2009). Excess heart-disease-related mortality in a national study of patients with mental disorders: identifying modifiable risk factors. *Gen Hosp Psychiatry*, **31**, 555–563.

17. Abdullah, H.M., Azeb Shahul, H., Hwang, M.Y., Ferrando, S. (2020). Comorbidity in schizophrenia: conceptual issues and clinical management. *Focus (Am Psychiatr Publ)*, **18**(4), 386–390. https://doi.org/10.1176/appi.focus.20200026

18. Hwang, M.Y., Nasrallah, H.A. (2009). Preface. *Psychiatr Clin N Am*, **32**(4), xiii–xv. https://doi.org/10.1016/j.psc.2009.10.002

19. Correll, C.U., Rubio, J.M., Inczedy-Farkas, G., et al. (2017). Efficacy of 42 pharmacologic cotreatment strategies added to antipsychotic monotherapy in schizophrenia: systematic overview and quality appraisal of the meta-analytic evidence. *JAMA Psychiatry*, **74**(7), 675–684.

20. Vancampfort, D., Correll, C.U., Galling, B., et al. (2016). Diabetes mellitus in people with schizophrenia, bipolar disorder and major depressive disorder: a systematic review and large scale meta-analysis. *World Psychiatry*, **15**(2), 166–174. https://doi.org/10.1002/wps.20309

21. Siris, S.G. (2001). Suicide and schizophrenia. *J Psychopharmacol*, **15**(2), 127–135. https://doi.org/10.1177/026988110101500209

22. National Institute for Health and Care Excellence. (2014). *Psychosis and schizophrenia in adults: prevention and management* [NICE Clinical Guideline GC178].

23. First, M.B., Gaebel, W., Maj, M., et al. (2021). An organization- and category-level comparison of diagnostic requirements for mental disorders in ICD-11 and DSM-5. *World Psychiatry*, **20**(1), 34–51. https://doi.org/10.1002/wps.20825

24. Jansson, L.B., Parnas, J. (2007). Competing definitions of schizophrenia: what can be learned from polydiagnostic studies? *Schizophr Bull*, **33**, 1178–1200.

25. Dixon, L.B., Goldman, H.H., Srihari, V.H., Kane, J.M. (2018). Transforming the treatment of schizophrenia in the United States: the RAISE initiative. *Annu Rev Clin Psychol*, **14**, 237–258.

26. Marneros, A., Tsuang, M.T. (2007). *Affective and Schizoaffective Disorders. Similarities and Differences*. New York: Springer Verlag. https://doi.org/10.1007/978-3-642-75353-4

27. Reed, G.M., Sharan, P., Rebello, T.J., et al. (2018). The ICD-11 developmental field study of reliability of diagnoses of high-burden mental disorders: results among adult patients in mental health settings of 13 countries. *World Psychiatry*, **17**(2), 174–186. https://doi.org/10.1002/wps.20524

28. Chmielewski, M., Clark, L.A., Bagby, R.M., Watson, D. (2015). Method matters: understanding diagnostic reliability in DSM-IV and DSM-5. *J Abnorm Psychol*, **124**(3), 764–769. https://doi.org/10.1037/abn0000069

29. Gaebel, W., Riesbeck, M., Zielasek, J., et al. (2018). [Web-based field studies on diagnostic classification and code assignment of mental disorders: comparison of ICD-11 and ICD-10]. *Fortschr Neurol Psychiatr*, **86**(3), 163–171. https://doi.org/10.1055/s-0044-100508

30. Gaebel, W., Stricker, J., Riesbeck, M., et al. (2020). Accuracy of diagnostic classification and clinical utility assessment of ICD-11 compared to ICD-10 in 10 mental disorders: findings from a web-based field study. *Eur Arch Psychiatry Clin Neurosci*, **270**(3), 281–289. https://doi.org/10.1007/s00406-019-01076-z

31. Stein, D.J., Szatmari, P., Gaebel, W., et al. (2020). Mental, behavioral and neurodevelopmental disorders in the ICD-11: an international perspective on key changes and controversies. *BMC Med*, **18**, 21. https://doi.org/10.1186/s12916-020-1495-2

32. Gaebel, W., Salveridou-Hof, E. (2022). Reinventing schizophrenia: updating the construct – primary schizophrenia 2021 – the road ahead. *Schizophr Res*, **242**, 27–29. https://doi.org/10.1016/j.schres.2021.12.021

Chapter 4

Mood Disorders

Gin S. Malhi & Erica Bell

Introductory Remarks

The first thing that is perhaps most. noticeable to those familiar with ICD-10 is that in ICD-11, the term 'affective' is no longer applied to the grouping of these disorders.[1] 'Mood disorders' now sits under the parent descriptor 'Mental, Behavioural or Neurodevelopmental Disorders' and subsumes both bipolar and depressive disorders. The consideration of mood disorders as a single group is consistent with ICD-10, but remains a key point of difference with DSM-5, where depressive and bipolar disorders have been set apart and are considered completely separately as 'Depressive disorders' and 'Bipolar and related disorders'. Notably, this is not a carry-over from DSM-IV, where in fact the two sets of disorders were considered together under the term 'Mood Disorders'.

In ICD-11, mood disorders are defined based on the types of mood episodes and their pattern over time. The episodes themselves are *not* independently diagnosable, and as such do not attract a diagnostic code. In other words, the episodes are components of the disorders, which therefore are the only diagnoses that can be coded and captured statistically. This is important because it means single or recurrent episodes of mania, and single or recurrent mixed episodes, if occurring outside the context of a depressive disorder, can only be captured under bipolar disorder (see further discussion below). The mood disorders are therefore constructed from several types of mood episodes: depressive, manic, mixed, and hypomanic (see Table 4.1). Combinations of these four kinds of episodes give rise to mood disorders, which include a *single episode depressive disorder*, *recurrent depressive disorder*, *dysthymic disorder*, and bipolar or related disorders that include *bipolar type I disorder*, *bipolar type II disorder*, *cyclothymic disorder*, and *other-specified bipolar or related disorders*.

Comments on Structure

It is 30 years since ICD-10 was released, and during the past decade ICD-11 has been in development, so the revision process has spanned the release of DSM-5 in 2013 and its subsequent uptake. And whilst one of its primary aims is to maintain continuity with its predecessor (ICD-10), ICD-11 has also attempted to some extent to harmonize its structure with DSM-5 and standardize descriptions to limit arbitrary differences. These attempts are evident in its mood disorders section. One of the key differences, however, is that ICD-11 aims for broader use in clinical practice across the world, in a variety of settings, as opposed

---

This chapter draws on elements of a virtual presentation at the 2021 Royal College of Psychiatrists Congress (UK) given by Professors Gin Malhi and Michael Berk, and a debate between Professors Gin Malhi and Andrew Nierenberg at the World Federation for Biological Psychiatry Congress in Vancouver (Canada) in 2019.

Table 4.1 ICD-11 Mood Disorders classification system

Mood Episodes	Depressive Disorders*	Bipolar or Related Disorders
Depressive episode	Single Episode Depressive Disorder	Bipolar Type I Disorder
Manic episode	Recurrent Depressive Disorder	Bipolar Type II Disorder
Mixed episode	Dysthymic Disorder	Cyclothymic Disorder
Hypomanic episode	Other Specified Depressive Disorders	Other Specified Bipolar or Related Disorders

* Mixed depressive and anxiety disorder is also included in the section on depressive disorders.
Note: Substance-induced Mood Disorder as a secondary mood syndrome is coded elsewhere and Premenstrual Dysphoric Disorder is classified within premenstrual disturbances under diseases of the genitourinary system. Where mood symptoms do not fulfil the diagnostic criteria for any of these mood disorders, then a diagnosis of other-specified mood disorder may be appropriate.

to DSM-5, which is primarily geared for use in the USA, where management is very much predicated on having a diagnosis listed in the *Diagnostic and Statistical Manual*. Consequently, the strict diagnostic criteria of DSM-5 are less evident in ICD-11, where features are described as *essential* and *required* but stringent symptom counts and duration cut-offs are not applied.[2] Clinicians are therefore afforded greater freedom to use their clinical judgement.

Depressive Episode

The clinical features of depression are divided into those that are *essential* (required) and those that are deemed *additional*. The essential features are further subdivided into three clusters: *affective*, *cognitive-behavioural*, and *neurovegetative* (see Figure 4.1). In total there are ten symptoms that are thought to be characteristic of a depressive episode. These must occur most of the day, nearly every day, during a period of at least 2 weeks, and at least five of these symptoms should be present concurrently. Furthermore, amongst these, at least one symptom should be from the affective cluster. The latter contains two symptoms – depressed mood and a markedly diminished interest or pleasure in activities (anhedonia). Interestingly, the marked decrease in interest or pleasure includes a reduction in sexual desire – an important symptom that is surprisingly often overlooked in clinical practice.[3] Further, the depressed mood can be reported subjectively or objectively, and in children and adolescents the depressive syndrome can manifest predominantly as irritability.

The *cognitive-behavioural* cluster contains four symptoms with indecisiveness added to reduced ability to concentrate and maintain attention to tasks, and beliefs about low self-worth (previously reduced self-esteem and self-confidence) are combined with excessive and inappropriate guilt that may be delusional. Importantly, it is specified that this item does not apply if the feelings of guilt or self-reproach are predominantly related to being depressed (i.e., they are mood congruent). Bleak and pessimistic views of the future are summed up as hopelessness, and ideas or acts of self-harm or suicide are expanded to include recurrent thoughts of death. Furthermore, recurrent suicidal ideation does not require a specific plan.

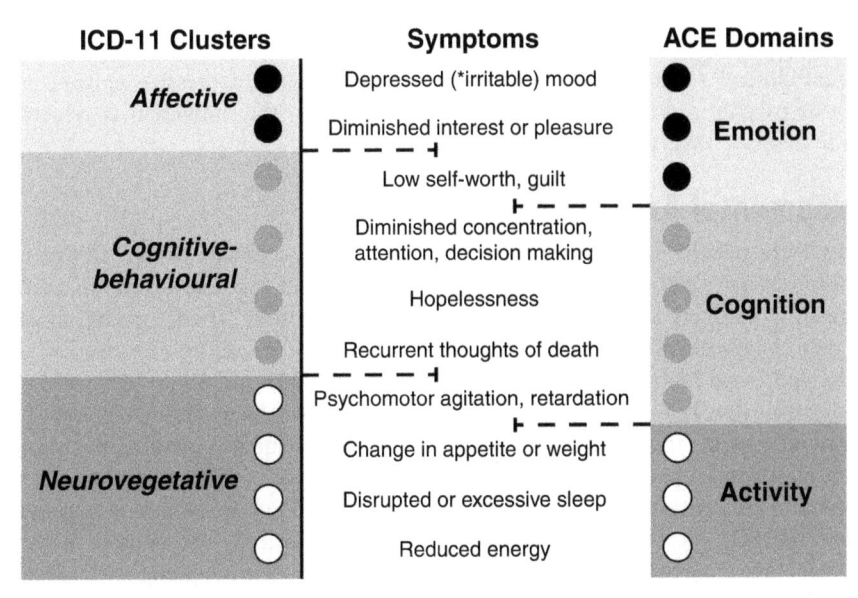

ICD-11 Clusters	Symptoms	ACE Domains
Affective ● ●	Depressed (*irritable) mood Diminished interest or pleasure	● ● Emotion
Cognitive-behavioural ○ ○ ○ ○	Low self-worth, guilt Diminished concentration, attention, decision making Hopelessness Recurrent thoughts of death	● ○ ○ Cognition ○
Neurovegetative ○ ○ ○ ○	Psychomotor agitation, retardation Change in appetite or weight Disrupted or excessive sleep Reduced energy	○ ○ ○ Activity ○

Figure 4.1 Symptoms of depression forming clusters in ICD-11 and domains in the ACE model.[4] The figure shows the typical symptoms of a depressive episode. These are grouped into clusters within ICD-11 and into domains that are dimensional constructs in the ACE model. The overlap between the two schemas is notable and within the ACE model hopelessness is aligned with suicidal ideation. It is also worth commenting that ACE emphasizes the cognitive components of psychomotor changes but attaches greater value to the emotional strands of guilt and worthlessness. It is important to note that in children and adolescents, the depressed mood can manifest as irritability (denoted by asterisk). Shaded circles indicate the symptom cluster to which each symptom belongs according to ICD-11 (affective = black, cognitive-behavioural = grey, neurovegetative = white) and according to the ACE (activity, cognition, and emotion) domain in which each symptom is predominant according to the ACE model (activity = white, cognition = grey, emotion = black).

The *neurovegetative cluster* also contains four symptoms and disrupted sleep is spelled out in greater detail, taking into consideration, for example, delay in onset, increased frequency of waking during the night, or early morning wakening. Similarly, appetite is now described as diminished or increased, or alternatively there can be significant weight change through gain or loss. Interestingly, changes in energy are included in this cluster along with fatigue and psychomotor changes (agitation or retardation) that have been made more explicit.

Additional Clinical Features

Notably, ICD-11 now includes irritability as a primary feature and, along with an absence of emotional experiences, described as 'emptiness', these two clinical features are seen as potential variants of the affective component and satisfy the mood requirement for a depressive episode if there is a significant change from typical functioning. This is particularly noteworthy, as irritability has been variably defined in both major taxonomies (ICD and DSM),[5] and still connotes different aspects of mood depending on age according to DSM-5 (see discussion).[6]

The absence of any emotional experience, described as an emptiness, is also noteworthy, and in addition to reflecting the fact that many patients with depression are unable to articulate their experience, it runs the risk of being confused with the more pervasive sense of emptiness sometimes found in patients with borderline personality disorder.[7] Other additional clinical features that are noted apply to a severe depressive episode where, because of psychotic symptoms or psychomotor changes, the individual is reluctant or unable to describe their experiences.

Developmental Aspects

Depressive episodes in ICD-11 are further characterized according to age. Depression is uncommon prior to puberty and appears to have no gender bias. However, after puberty, girls are twice as likely as boys to develop a depressive episode.[8] Furthermore, in adolescence, depressive episodes are similar to those experienced by adults. However, in young children, depressed mood may present as somatic complaints and other symptoms within the affective cluster. Pervasive irritability is also perhaps more likely, though in and of itself, it is not necessarily indicative of a depressive episode. Equally, within the cognitive-behavioural cluster, special consideration should be given to differentiate problems of attention and concentration to distinguish depression from attention deficit hyperactivity disorder (ADHD), an important differential diagnosis. Critically, depression in children and adolescents is associated with an increased risk of suicidality, along with other self-injurious behaviours.

Severity and Psychotic Symptoms Specifiers

The ICD-11 retains its emphasis on severity, based on the number of symptoms and their impact on functioning. Episodes are therefore described as *mild*, *moderate*, and *severe*, with moderate and severe episodes further specified as with or without psychotic symptoms. This is much the same as ICD-10, except that now moderate depressive episodes can also have psychotic symptoms coded. This is important as it speaks to the increasing recognition of the dimensionality of mood symptoms and disorders (see discussion).

Comments on ICD-11 Depressive Episodes

In ICD-11, a diagnosis of depression is possible in the context of bereavement following a major adverse event such as divorce or death. However, the threshold for a depressive episode is now extended in duration from 2 weeks to at least 1 month, indicating a persistence of depressive symptoms, during which time there should be no periods of positive mood or enjoyment of activities. Furthermore, symptoms of low self-worth and guilt and extreme beliefs that are not related to loss are more indicative of depression in the context of bereavement, as are unusual and characteristic features such as suicidal ideation, psychotic symptoms, or psychomotor retardation. When attempting to distinguish depression and bereavement, a prior history of depression also clearly suggests the likelihood of a recurrence. Nevertheless, it is important to emphasize that depression should *not* be confused with normal grief symptoms, and that following the death of a loved one, it is to be expected that an individual will experience symptoms that give the impression of the individual being depressed.

Six months' duration is provided as a broad guide to diagnosis, given that cultural and religious considerations will also impact on both the severity and duration of 'normal' grief and it should be noted that grief and bereavement are not especially prone to arise in future depression. Thus, in ICD-11, a diagnosis of depression can be superimposed on normal grief and in contrast to DSM-5, where the differentiation is largely based on clinical judgement, in ICD-11 more careful consideration is given to the *nature* of the symptoms, their *severity* and *duration*.

Manic Episode

The other key episode within mood disorders that defines the various types of disorders is mania. Interestingly, mania does not have a separate status as an entity as does depression (e.g., recurrent depressive episodes are captured as a depressive disorder), and recurrent manic episodes do not constitute a 'manic disorder' analogous to depressive disorder. Instead, they are subsumed within bipolar disorder, which encompasses depressive episodes. But clinically, unipolar mania *is* a separate entity (see discussion later) and research to date warrants its consideration, both clinically and for future research and investigation, as a distinct disorder.

The features of mania in ICD-11 have approximated further towards those specified in DSM-5 (see Figure 4.2). ICD-11 lists essential features (those that are required) and specifies two principal features that need to occur concurrently and persist for most of the day, nearly every day, during a period of at least 1 week (unless this period is shortened by a treatment intervention).

The first of these features is an extreme mood state that can be characterized by euphoria, irritability, or expansiveness (all of these are a significant departure from the individual's usual mood). Further, it is noted that rapid changes among the different mood states often occur, and these are described as mood lability.

Activity
Increased energy*
Decreased need for sleep
Impulsive, reckless behaviour
Increased sexual drive, sociability, goal-directed activity

Cognition
Increased talkativeness, pressured speech
Increased self-esteem, grandiosity
Distractibility

Emotion
Extreme mood* – euphoria, irritability, expansiveness, mood lability
Flight of ideas, rapid or racing thoughts

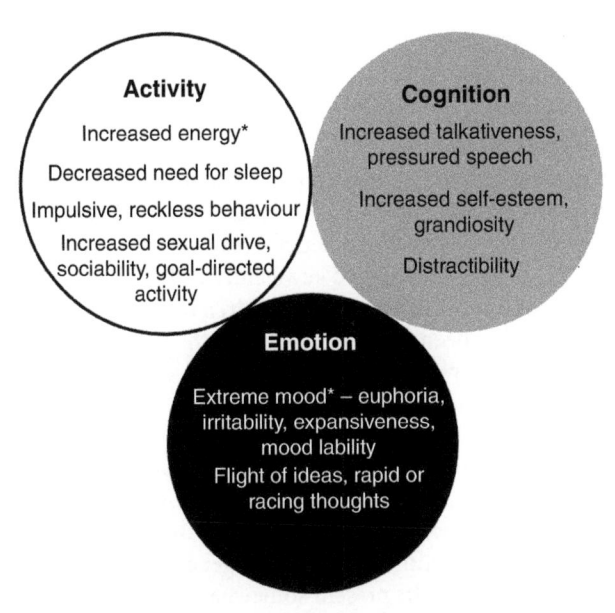

Figure 4.2 Features of a manic episode in ICD-11. This schematic illustrates how the features of a manic episode in ICD-11 can be grouped according to the domains outlined in the ACE model (activity, cognition, and emotion). The essential features of a manic episode include both increased energy and extreme mood (denoted by an asterisk).

The second feature is that of increased activity or a subjective experience of heightened energy, and again this a significant change from the individual's normal levels of energy and activity. These features are essentially those of criterion A in a manic episode in DSM-5, but whereas DSM-5 specifies three or more additional symptoms (four if the mood is only irritable), ICD-11 simply states 'several', which essentially means 'more than two and fewer than many'. In other words, ICD-11 means three or more from a list of seven.

The descriptive approach to bipolar disorder is more apparent in ICD-11, as it is subsumed under mood disorders, and either a manic episode or mixed episode is sufficient for a diagnosis of bipolar disorder. The duration criterion for mania is at least 1 week and while this is the same as DSM-5, and indeed for DSM-IV and ICD-10, it remains a problem when considering mixed episodes (see later).

Naturally, the clinical presentation of a manic episode should not fulfil the diagnostic requirements for a mixed episode, even though a wide variety of symptoms can occur in mania including psychotic symptoms. Most commonly, the latter are grandiose delusions, but delusions of a persecutory or self-referential nature and those relating to experiences of passivity can also occur, as can delusions that thoughts are being placed in one's mind (thought insertion) or withdrawn, or that they are being broadcast to others. However, these are unusual, as are hallucinations, and if hallucinations do occur, they are usually in keeping with the mood state and are often adulatory. Importantly, it has been noted that if the symptom requirements satisfy the diagnosis of a manic episode, then this is the diagnosis that should be made even if, because of treatment, the duration criterion is not met. In other words, because of the urgency of treating mania, it is common to prescribe sedating medications that may remove or mask most symptoms almost immediately. Consequently, is not unusual for a 'manic episode' to technically last only a matter of a few days as opposed to a full week. In these instances, ICD-11 allows coding for such an episode as mania. Another way of thinking about this is that the severity of the symptoms and their number are regarded as more important than duration per se.

Developmental Aspects

The occurrence of mania is rare in children and adolescents. ICD-11 describes it as 'normal' for children to express exuberance, silliness, or over-excitement. Furthermore, to qualify for mania, ICD-11 suggests that all the characteristic features of a manic episode should be apparent. However, it is quite likely that the key feature is that of extreme irritability rather than a change in mood per se, and in very young children this may manifest as tantrums and physical aggression. There has been much debate about the status of the diagnosis of mania in young people and especially in children. As such, a diagnosis of paediatric bipolar disorder remains contentious (see discussion).[9-11]

Another potential area for confusion is distractibility, which in children may result in a decline in academic performance and an inability to complete assignments on time. This can cause problems in separating bipolar disorder from ADHD. Further, grandiosity is difficult to define in children, and it is normal for them to overestimate their abilities or believe that they have special talents or powers. In general, many of the symptoms that characterize a manic episode in adults present somewhat differently in younger age groups, and therefore these must be judged depending on the level of development of the child or adolescent and their context.

Boundaries and Differential Diagnosis for a Manic Episode

A key diagnostic distinction within the manic spectrum is that between a hypomanic and a manic episode. A potential differentiator seems to be the degree of impairment in personal, family, social, educational, and occupational functioning, and these domains are affected to a greater extent in a manic episode. However, the other criteria that are said to differentiate hypomania and mania are arguably less valid and have been debated, such as the need for hospitalization and the duration of symptoms (see Parker and Malhi[12,13]).

Mania also overlaps with mixed episodes, and indeed, up until recently most mixed episodes were subsumed within mania for the purposes of clinical trials. This is because, in practice, mania seems to trump depression, in that the emergence of manic symptoms transmutes a diagnosis of depression to bipolar disorder (see discussion later). Similarly, greater credence and value are attached to manic symptoms, and, therefore, in a mixed episode in which depressive symptoms are regarded as subsidiary, the episode is more likely to be branded as a manic episode. However, ICD-11 has now developed criteria specifically for a mixed episode (see below).

Another overlap discussed in ICD-11 is that between a manic episode and ADHD. The potential for confusion arises because both feature increased activity, rapid speech, impulsivity, and distractibility. Therefore, separating the two in children and adolescents is particularly difficult, although symptoms of ADHD usually emerge before the age of 12 and persist over time. In other words, they are not related to changes in mood or energy, and indeed mood is not a prominent feature and in general the symptoms are not episodic. Again, this has proven to be a difficult diagnostic distinction, and as a consequence, there is much debate as to the real prevalence of both ADHD and bipolar disorder and their overlap, especially in young people.[9]

Comments on ICD-11 Manic Episode

As noted earlier, in both ICD-11 and DSM-5, a diagnosis of bipolar disorder requires an essential feature of increased energy or activity. This is in addition to either elated, euphoric, expansive, or irritable mood, and this requirement is a significant departure from their respective predecessors (ICD-10 and DSM-IV), which only require the presence of criterion A, namely, mood changes. The centrality of energy is in keeping with the ACE model (activity, cognition, and emotion), and we have discussed the importance of energy both for clinical practice and for understanding the mechanisms of mood disorders. For example, it is postulated that a core disturbance of energy, perhaps within mitochondria, is at the heart of the pathophysiology of bipolar disorder.[14]

Hypomanic Episode

The clinical features for a hypomanic episode are essentially the same as those for a manic episode; however, the wording describing hypomania in ICD-11 is slightly different, and some additional aspects are thought to separate the two presentations. Like mania, the clinical features in hypomania should be present for most of the day, nearly every day, but the overall duration of the episode is only several days rather than at least a week. Furthermore, whereas in mania the mood state is described as 'extreme', in hypomania the emphasis is more on persistence. For a manic episode, the significant change has to be distinguishable from the individual's 'typical mood'; however, for hypomania the comparator is 'usual range of moods' and does not include those that are contextually appropriate. Again, in addition to these key symptoms, there are several additional essential features, and these are the same as those for mania. Naturally, the episode should not meet requirements for mania and nor indeed a mixed episode. Importantly, the mood disturbance should not be so severe as to cause marked impairment in occupational functioning, or in usual social activities, or relationships with others, and is not accompanied by delusions or hallucinations. This then is a key distinction between mania and hypomania, where the former results in significant impairment, may require intensive treatment, and may be accompanied by delusions or hallucinations. However, like mania, a hypomanic syndrome can arise during antidepressant treatment, and, according to ICD-11, can be considered a hypomanic episode if it persists after the treatment is discontinued and the full diagnostic requirements are met.

Interestingly, the boundary with normality is more difficult, given that there is no significant functional impairment in hypomania, and it is accepted that brief changes in any of the typical symptoms of mania may occur as part of the normal vicissitudes of life, and in particular, elevated mood is understandable in the context of positive life events. Interestingly, the occurrence of hypomanic episodes in the absence of a history of other types of mood episodes, namely, mania, depression, or mixed episodes, is insufficient for a diagnosis of a mood disorder. This, therefore, distinguishes hypomania while also diminishing its significance.

Developmental Considerations

The developmental considerations for hypomania are similar to those for mania, as are the boundary considerations. The distinction with a manic episode, however, rests largely on severity and impairment, as the symptoms themselves are qualitatively similar (see above).

Mixed Episode

The definition of a mixed episode in ICD-11 is especially interesting and therefore worthy of detailed consideration. The essential features require the presence of several prominent manic and depressive symptoms, and these should be in keeping with those found in a manic or depressive episode (see previous). Curiously, they can occur simultaneously, or alternate rapidly from day to day or even within the same day. Key among these is an altered mood state that is consistent with a manic and/or depressive episode, in other words, depressed, dysphoric, euphoric, or expansive mood. This needs to be present most of the day, nearly every day during a period of at least 2 weeks.[1] Characterizing these further, ICD-11 states that when manic symptoms predominate in a mixed episode, the depressive symptoms (described as contra polar) usually include dysphoric mood, expressed beliefs of worthlessness, hopelessness, and suicidal ideation (see Figure 4.3). Conversely, when depressive symptoms predominate in a mixed episode, the common contra polar manic symptoms include irritability, racing or crowded thoughts, increased talkativeness, and increased activity. Notably, no specific number of symptoms is specified. ICD-11 further allows alternate rapid cycling during a mixed episode between depressive and manic symptoms and describes these as fluctuations that may be observed in mood, emotional reactivity, drive, and cognitive function.

---

[1] Unless shortened by a treatment intervention.

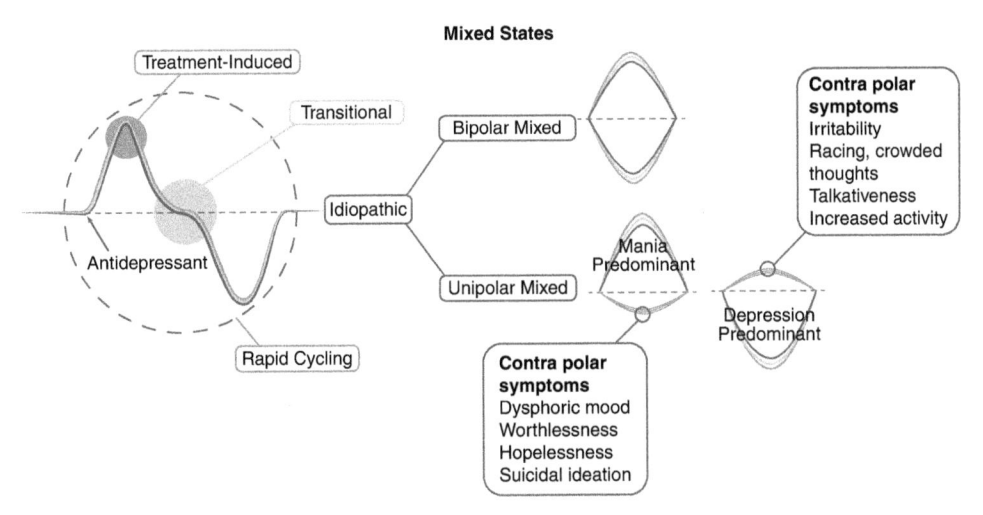

Figure 4.3 Overview of mixed states as classified in ICD-11. In ICD-11, the essential features of a mixed state include several prominent manic and depressive symptoms. These can be treatment-induced (e.g., due to an antidepressant), can occur when *transitioning* from a manic to a depressive episode (or vice versa), and can seem to occur because of *rapid cycling* between the two mood states. The distribution of the manic and depressive symptoms can be even (bipolar mixed) or either mania or depression can predominate (unipolar mixed), with contra polar symptoms creating an admixture.

As with other episodes, the symptoms should not be manifestations of another medical condition or because of the effects of a substance or medication. The mood disturbance overall should result in significant impairment and impact a number of areas of functioning, or be accompanied by delusions or hallucinations. Given that both depressive and manic symptoms feature in mixed episodes, the delusions and hallucinations also reflect the content of both depression and mania. Furthermore, in line with mania, a mixed syndrome that arises during antidepressant treatment is to be considered a mixed episode if it persists after the treatment is discontinued and the diagnostic requirements of a mixed episode have been met. Thus, the description of a mixed episode in ICD-11 is starkly different to that in DSM-5.

Dysthymic Disorder

Dysthymic disorder in ICD-11 refers to what is commonly called dysthymia. This is experienced by patients as predominantly low mood that is present for most of the time, over a period of at least 2 years (see Figure 4.4). Critically, during this period, at no point should the severity of symptoms meet the criteria for a depressive episode. Typical symptoms of dysthymia, which is in essence a sub-syndromal form of depression, include anhedonia, low self-esteem, guilt, impaired concentration, pessimism, and disturbed sleep and appetite with prolonged periods of fatigue. Notably, dysthymia does not have the significant impairment that is characteristic of depressive episodes and major depressive disorder. Dysthymia is also devoid of suicidality and symptoms such as psychomotor retardation and agitation. Naturally, there should be no symptoms of mania at any point in time. Thus, the key factors that differentiate dysthymia from depression are the degree of functional impairment and the severity of symptoms over an extended period.

Persistent Depressive Disorder

In DSM-5, dysthymic disorder is described as persistent depressive disorder (PDD). As outlined already, many of the features are consistent with a chronic depressive episode that is sometimes confusingly referred to as a 'depressive personality'. Like dysthymia, PDD lasts more than 2 years and consists of depressed mood with features of low energy, fatigue, changes in sleep and appetite, low self-esteem, poor concentration, and indecisiveness and hopelessness. Notably, a period of 2 months (continuous) during which there are no symptoms excludes a diagnosis of PDD. In other words, continuity must be maintained. Another distinction from dysthymic disorder in ICD-11 is that if the full criteria for major depressive disorder are met and have been present continuously for a period of more than 2 years, then a diagnosis of PDD can still be made (see Figure 4.4). This is the reason in DSM-5 that PDD includes patients with severe functional impairment. In other words, PDD is very different to dysthymic disorder, and it can commence in adolescence.

Cyclothymic Disorder

Like dysthymia, cyclothymic disorder in ICD-11 also has a duration of 2 years or more. During this time, an individual may experience multiple symptoms of hypomania and symptoms of dysthymia, but none of these periods should reach the threshold for a formal depressive episode or indeed a manic episode. Cyclothymia therefore subsumes periods of hypomania that are not accompanied by depressive episodes. Further, in contrast to dysthymia, in ICD-11 the symptoms of cyclothymic disorder may produce significant impairment of function, and while a manic episode would transmute the diagnosis to bipolar I disorder, the existence of hypomanic episodes, along with a prolonged period of unstable mood, does *not* confer a diagnosis of bipolar II disorder. Instead, it would require an additional depressive episode to reach the threshold for bipolar II as defined in ICD-11. Interestingly, cyclothymic disorder is similar in both DSM-5 and ICD-11; however, it does not require marked or significant impairment of functioning, which allows more moderate presentations to be included.

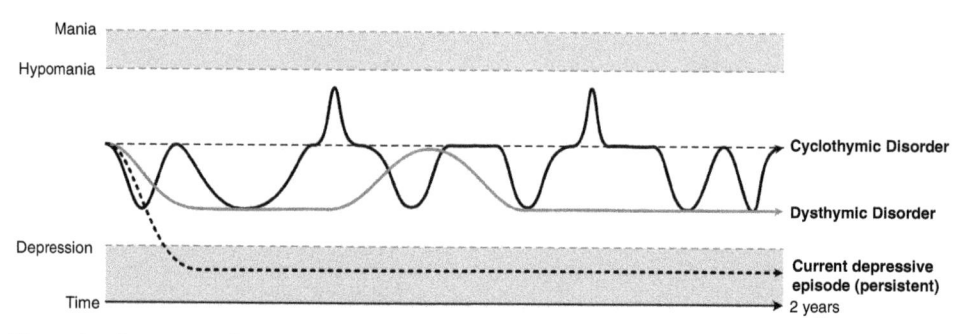

Figure 4.4 Comparison of diagnostic criteria for cyclothymic disorder, dysthymic disorder, and current depressive episode (persistent) according to ICD-11. This schematic shows that both dysthymic disorder (grey line) and cyclothymic disorder (black line) entail less severe/subsyndromal mood symptoms that do not meet the threshold for a hypomanic/manic or depressive episode but persist for at least 2 years. In contrast, a persistent episode of depression (dotted line) entails meeting the threshold for a depressive episode, and for this to then persist over a period of 2 years, during which time it can incur significant functional impairment.

Discussion

Having outlined the structure of the ICD-11 mood disorder section and some of the key disorders defined using combinations of the various kinds of mood episodes, in conjunction with qualifiers such as duration of illness and degree of impairment, we now compare some sections with ICD-10 and DSM-5 and discuss the clinical implications of the differences.

One of the tensions that arises in any classificatory system concerning diseases that is perhaps more prominent when considering mental disorders is recognizing that individual symptoms and syndromes are on a continuum, and that across the human experience they form a spectrum that does not necessarily provide clear markers as to where an illness begins as it departs from normality. This problem of having to impose categories for the purposes of labelling, treating, and collecting data for epidemiological purposes and other forms of research means that diagnostic categories are often an approximation of clinical reality. In other words, the boundaries of disorders and diagnoses are often fuzzy. This difficulty is particularly evident in mood disorders where anxiety, a normal phenomenon, is often admixed with depressive symptoms which are, by and large, aberrations of normal experience (e.g., reduced sleep). A further problem is that the phenomenology of mood disorders comprises both objective and subjective symptoms and that ironically mood, the term that is used to define the whole group of disorders, while exquisitely sensitive is probably the least specific for these disorders. As a consequence, it has only modest discriminant value and places a disproportionate burden on other symptoms with respect to diagnostic differentiation.

Commentary and Critique

Having highlighted the key changes in ICD-11, it's important to comment more specifically on where things have changed in relation to ICD-10 and compare these changes to ICD-11's counterpart, namely, DSM-5. Where possible, some of these similarities and differences have been pointed out in the foregoing text, when describing the criteria for various episodes; however, this section examines a number of contentious diagnoses that have attracted extensive discussion and therefore warrant further scrutiny. Note, for each of these, references have been provided for further reading for those interested in delving deeper into various controversies. Therefore, in this chapter, only the main points are covered, and since we have contributed ourselves actively to some of these discussions, we declare from the outset our personal bias in presenting this material.

The Symptoms of Mood Disorders

The ICD-11 considers both depressive and bipolar disorders under the one heading of mood disorders, which recognizes their commonalities and, in particular, the fact that depression spans both sets of disorders. There are also many commonalities in aetiological factors, and a significant number of treatments are shared. This is the principal reason as to why the Royal Australian and New Zealand College of Psychiatrists (RANZCP) guidelines addressed the management of mood disorders jointly as opposed to having individual depressive and bipolar disorders guidelines.[15] Another development in ICD-11 that we support is the use of clusters to group the various symptoms within depression. The affective, cognitive-behavioural, and neurovegetative clusters provide a useful subgrouping of the symptoms and shift the focus away from mood symptoms to other domains. This is particularly important in mania, where energy, for example, an activity symptom, is arguably more characteristic of the syndrome and perhaps even deserves primacy. These clusters are very much in keeping with our proposal for the ACE model, which comprises activity, cognition, and emotion (tallies broadly with neurovegetative, cognitive-behavioural, and affective). The ACE model, which we have outlined in detail elsewhere,[4] provides continuity across the various mood disorders and readily accommodates mixed states. It also explains treatment-induced changes in mood such as treatment-emergent mania and provides a more nuanced understanding of the composition of mood disorders.

Unfortunately, in ICD-11, the clusters have only been applied to depressive episodes, even though the mood disorders that would perhaps benefit most from such a framework are mixed states and bipolar disorders. Nevertheless, there are hints that ICD-11 has taken a more dimensional approach in general, for example making suggestions as to which symptoms to look for and nominating these as 'several' rather than specifying numbers and setting thresholds. This places greater responsibility on clinicians but at the same time allows greater freedom for clinical judgement. However, while this is advantageous for clinical practice, it is not an approach that can be readily applied to research questions and therefore DSM-5 is likely to retain its dominance in this regard.

One clear signal that ICD-11 regards the mood disorders more as a spectrum than DSM-5 is the inclusion of mixed episodes. This was removed from DSM-5, in part because of its under-utility in DSM-IV. A major reason for its neglect was its poor definition, which necessitated that both sets of symptoms of depression and mania be present in full, and concurrently. This was very limiting, and it did not reflect clinical reality. However, unfortunately, DSM-5 has overcompensated and relegated mixed episodes to 'features' that are now only recognized as a specifier. This means that mixed symptoms can only be captured in the context of a depressive or manic episode, and the richness of mixed presentations has been lost. Thankfully, this is not the case in ICD-11, which does still allow for mixed episodes to be coded (quite correctly). However, because of the difference in duration between a depressive episode and an episode of mania (at least 2 weeks and 1 week, respectively), it is unclear how the different kinds of mixed presentations will be further disentangled so as to examine the nature of mixed states.

Bipolar II Disorder

The comments made above concerning capturing dimensional constructs and attempting to partition them, and the difficulties therein, are exemplified by the diagnosis of bipolar II disorder. This diagnosis was created following the observations of Dunner and colleagues.[16] They had noted different outcomes in patients depending on their mood state at the time of presentation. Patients admitted when depressed fared differently to those who presented with mania. To differentiate the two, they were labelled as type I and type II, and as manic-depressive illness presentations were examined in different contexts, a somewhat modified proposal emerged to incorporate bipolar subtypes into DSM.

The concept of subtyping is completely logical, and the initial aims were in keeping with the framework suggested by Robins and Guze,[17] that is, to further examine and investigate various disorders so as to find explanatory models and underpinnings that would inform treatment and management. However, bipolar II disorder has remained firmly within the realm of phenomenology.[12] As pointed out above when discussing the changes to ICD-11, the distinction between a hypomanic episode and a manic episode is arbitrary with regard to the duration of symptoms. The need for hospitalization is a unique specifier, which in modern-day practice is largely meaningless. Psychosis is somewhat helpful but only if modelled dimensionally, and similarly impairment is meaningful but, again, difficult to assess, somewhat subjective, and challenging to standardize. Thus, after 40 years, surely ample opportunity has been provided to identify the substrates for bipolar II disorder. Alas, no new insights have been forthcoming, and therefore the model should be set aside[13] – especially as it is increasingly apparent that manic symptoms can and do last for shorter periods of time than 4 days and that there is no trend break in terms of treatment or other phenomenology between a manic episode of 2 days and those lasting longer. An in-depth discussion of this matter can be found in recent viewpoints.[12,13]

It is somewhat disappointing that ICD-11 has adopted bipolar II disorder as part of its taxonomy. This is despite the fact that, in practice, it has been shown to overlap considerably and consistently with personality disorder.[18] Furthermore, confusion is common when diagnosing bipolar disorder and ADHD in youth.[9] More generally, the introduction of bipolar II disorder has increased the diagnosis of bipolar disorder and increased the likelihood of masking those with other sets of problems. However, at the same time, the changes to the core criteria of mania, namely, the inclusion of increased energy and activity alongside mood and/or irritability, will probably raise the threshold for bipolar disorder, and thereby push some patients towards depression. In this regard, an advantage of the ICD-11 descriptor for mania and bipolar II disorder is that there is no lower cut-off, and 'several days' can be interpreted as 3 days or more as opposed to the specified 4 days in DSM-5. Furthermore, the number of listed features is not pinned down, with the only suggestion being that 'several of the following' should be present. In contrast, DSM-5 requires at least three symptoms and specifies this, and so once again ICD-11 may allow greater flexibility.

Perhaps the most important consideration is what this will mean for treatment, and here it is clear that there are no specific treatments for so-called bipolar II disorder, just as there are no clear markers distinguishing it in terms of clinical course and outcome. This is the principal reason why the RANZCP mood disorders guidelines have made recommendations for bipolar disorders as a whole and across the board,[15] and most clinicians when asked feel comfortable simply transposing treatments from bipolar I disorder to manage cases of putative bipolar II. Finally, it is important to note that the few subtle differences that do exist, such as the predominance of depression in bipolar II as compared to bipolar I, are readily explained when the subtypes are placed dimensionally along the same spectrum.

Mixed Mood States

Embedded deep within the foundations of our current mood disorders taxonomy is a problem that surfaces daily, but we choose to ignore it. In 1899, Weygandt identified mixed mood states that were incorporated by Kraepelin into his classificatory schema.[19,20] These were based on domains of activity, cognition, and emotion (although different terms were used), and combinations of these allowed for two pure states of depression and mania and six states that were essentially 'admixtures'. This picture was drawn with patients in mind, as it best captured the clinical reality that Weygandt, Kraepelin, and their contemporaries observed. In addition to examining a broad range of symptoms across a number of domains, the approach also required adopting a longitudinal perspective. However, this was detailed and time-consuming and did not fit with the DSM approach. As a consequence, mixed states were constricted and eventually lost altogether.

In successive iterations of DSM, greater importance was placed on cross-sectional diagnoses with increasing focus on subtyping depression and mania, rather than examining the complexities of their intermingling. However, the clinical reality of patients with severe mood disorders has not changed, and at least a third of patients manifest mixed mood states. These mixed mood presentations are important, as they confer significant burden and are difficult to treat. They are associated with high levels of suicide and are frequently misdiagnosed. Thankfully, ICD-11 has maintained *mixed episodes*, albeit with rather relaxed definitions. Nevertheless, this is still significantly better than the system employed by DSM-5, which lacks logic and is likely to generate further confusion.

In DSM-5, mixed mood symptoms are denoted by a specifier that is attached to a mood episode. To qualify as a specifier, three or more symptoms from the opposite pole are needed. These are not nominated, and key symptoms such as irritability,[5,21] distractibility, and psychomotor changes are not attached any additional weight. Furthermore, there is no consideration given to any longitudinal pattern and symptoms are not grouped according to domains of activity, cognition, or emotion. In this regard, ICD-11 is considerably better, but puzzlingly the symptom clusters used to group depressive symptoms are not applied to the manic symptoms, which are essentially a reciprocal set (see Figure 4.2). One of the reasons DSM-5 has difficulty in accommodating mixed states, and to some extent this problem also applies to ICD-11, is that depressive and manic episodes are fundamentally seen as being mutually exclusive entities that are distinct and separate, and hence 'bipolar'. But in reality, the symptoms, syndromes, and indeed the disorders lie on a spectrum and comprise dimensional constructs. The ACE model alluded to previously captures this dimensionality and explains mixed states and also explains how treatment with an antidepressant intervention can induce manic symptoms (see Figure 4.5). Thus, while it is heartening to see that ICD-11 does have the ability to at least code mixed episodes, the fact that these are poorly specified and there is no continuity between the clusters in depression through to mania means that mixed states will remain difficult to capture and further advancement in our understanding of mixed mood states will prove challenging.

Personality Disorders

One section in which ICD-11 has adopted a dimensional approach and abandoned categorical classifications is that of personality disorders.[22] The key criterion is duration and symptoms are present for 2 years. During this time, the individual has a negative view of themselves (their self) or impaired interpersonal functioning, which essentially means dissatisfaction with their relationships or ongoing interpersonal conflict.[23] The upshot of this is dysfunctional behaviour that may impact a number of situations (such as personal life and workplace interactions). It may also result in distressing and maladaptive ways of thinking, along with disrupted emotional experiences involving emotional lability and dysregulation. All of this needs to meet the threshold of causing substantial distress or significant impairment in terms of functioning in order to attract a diagnosis of personality disorder.

Clearly, some of these symptoms, such as the dysregulation of emotional experiences, will have significant overlap with mood disorders.[24] The need for significant impairment, however, separates personality disorder from dysthymic disorder to some extent, but in clinical practice this may be difficult to determine. Similarly, there is considerable overlap with bipolar II disorder (see above). In particular, hypomanic episodes as defined by ICD-11

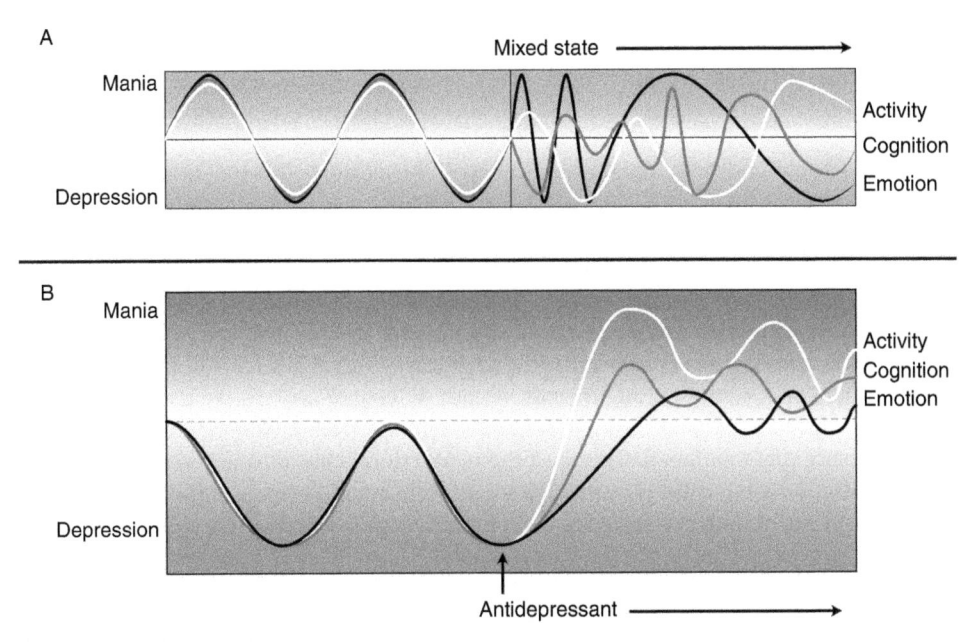

Figure 4.5 Mixed mood states. (A) How the ACE model conceptualizes mixed mood states as an uncoupling of symptoms within each of the domains of activity (white), cognition (grey), and emotion (black). When these symptoms are synchronized, they appear as unipolar depression or mania; however, uncoupling of the symptoms and domains produces a mixed mood state. (B) The effect of an antidepressant, which can lead to the uncoupling of the domains and thus produce a mixed state. The differential impact of an antidepressant – for example, affecting activity more than emotion and cognition – may lead to a difference emerging in the rate of change of symptoms such that the various domains are uncoupled for a period of time. This is a treatment-induced mixed state, which is different to an intrinsic (idiopathic) mixed state (see Figure 4.3).

will often include symptoms such as impulsivity, reckless behaviour, and irritability. These symptoms would also comfortably fit under the description of personality disorder as 'poorly regulated emotional expression and behaviour'. Thus, ultimately, the distinction between personality dysfunction and mood disorder falls to the clinician, and perhaps this is not a bad thing given the question marks surrounding the diagnosis of bipolar II disorder (see above). The chronicity of personality disorder necessitates a longitudinal and in-depth examination, because the nature of affective instability is different to that of changes in mood. The latter typically vary over a period of hours and days as opposed to changes in affect that vary over seconds and minutes. In addition, in personality disorders, there are many more complex psychosocial issues and relational issues to take into consideration, and thus having a clinician at the helm is invaluable. And while a lot of effort has been expended in trying to differentiate personality disorders from mood disorders, it is important to note that the two are not mutually exclusive and that in many cases they co-occur.

Mood Disorders in Youth

Understandably, there has been a longstanding desire to learn from where mood disorders emanate. Biological determinants seem likely, as do psychosocial factors and the environment as a whole, but piecing together the very many components has been difficult. This perhaps reflects the heterogeneity of the illnesses and indeed their inherent complexity. With increasing knowledge, it has become clearer that most mood disorders often first manifest in youth, and therefore concerted efforts are underway to detect and diagnose mood disorders in adolescence. And while most clinicians remain cautious when making a diagnosis in young people, there has been a growing interest over the past two decades in assigning mood disorders diagnoses to young adolescents and even prepubertal children. Predictably, this has been a source of immense contention and debate, and many of the controversies remain undecided.[10,25,11]

Perhaps as a response to the many discussions and debates that took place in the first decade of this century concerning over-diagnosis of mood disorders in youth, changes were made to DSM-5 and a totally new disorder, namely, disruptive mood dysregulation disorder (DMDD), was introduced. However, this diagnosis is also proving difficult and contentious,[26] and if nothing else this underscores the fact that the diagnosis of mood disorders in young people is difficult. Therefore, what is most urgently needed is longitudinal research that maps the trajectory of early behavioural disturbances and symptoms from childhood through puberty and adolescence into adulthood. This is all the more critical currently, as few treatments are available specifically for children and adolescents with mood symptoms/disorders, and the long-term benefits of both psychological and pharmacological therapies are unknown.

Conclusion

The diagnosis of a mood disorder is a critical step, and one that is usually undertaken by a psychiatrist or primary care physician. It is an important step, as it signifies a departure from normality and may indicate the need for treatment. It sets an individual on a particular course and, therefore, it is essential that the diagnosis be made with confidence so that a reasonable trajectory can be mapped. Mood disorders are complicated by their very nature, and separation from normal experiences and behaviour is often difficult and compounded further by the complexities of development, psychosocial context, and potential comorbidities. Nevertheless, diagnosis is essential, and ICD-11 provides a useful framework for clinicians. Still, researchers are likely to refer more to DSM-5, and possibly Research Domain Criteria (RDOC) (although this system is fast losing credibility) because these frameworks are more structured and adopt a more standardized and granular approach to both clarifying and understanding the substrates of disorders. However, a key perspective that is useful to all approaches is that of conducting assessments longitudinally, as mood disorders don't simply manifest but emerge gradually, and as they do so, they often evolve and transform (see Figure 4.6). A good example of this, which highlights to some extent the shortcomings of cross-sectional diagnoses, is the fact that most patients with bipolar disorder first develop a depressive episode. This may, however, begin with subsyndromal symptoms. and if detected, this would be diagnosed as dysthymia, provided, of course, that the symptoms have been present for more than 2 years. Once a depressive episode occurs, a diagnosis of major depression can be made, and if further episodes occur, as is often the case, then a recurrent major depression diagnosis is assigned. Treatment for this is prescribed accordingly; however, if the individual has an underlying bipolar illness, then at some point they will manifest manic symptoms. These may first emerge in the context of depression and may in fact be exacerbated by ongoing antidepressant treatment for the depressive symptoms. An astute clinician may well detect and diagnose a mixed episode; however, more than likely, these symptoms, and even those of mania if they are mild (hypomania in ICD-11), may be missed altogether. This is not uncommon and wholly

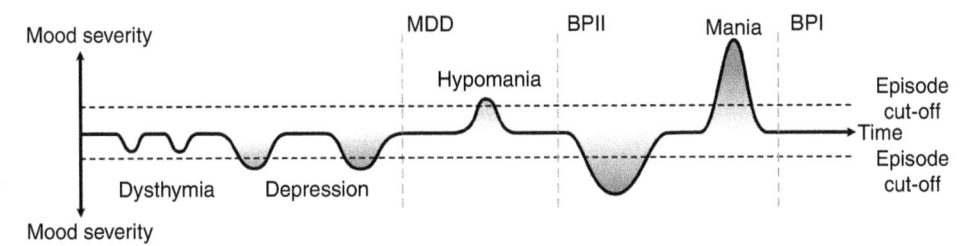

Figure 4.6 Diagnosis of mood episodes and disorders over time. This schematic shows the typical chronology of mood episodes in individuals with mood disorders. Subsyndromal depressive symptoms emerge first, which may, if sustained and accurately detected, attract a diagnosis of *dysthymia*. Following this, depressive symptoms may become more pronounced and form depressive episodes that then warrant a diagnosis of *major depressive disorder* (MDD). If the individual then subsequently experiences manic symptoms that satisfy the criteria for a hypomanic episode, a diagnosis of *bipolar II disorder* (BPII) could be assigned according to ICD-11. If these manic symptoms increase in severity and are more sustained, then a diagnosis of *bipolar I disorder* (BPI) may be assigned. In this way, an individual may 'accurately' meet the diagnostic requirements for several mood disorders over an extended period of time as symptoms emerge, evolve, and then manifest and fluctuate in severity – spanning the full spectrum of mood. Because of this natural history, the diagnosis of mood disorders is often subject to change, especially early in the course of illness.

understandable, given that mild manic symptoms are often enjoyable and may even be seemingly productive. If occurring in adolescence, they may be subsumed within the normal exuberance of youth or may be masked by the misuse of substances such as alcohol. Feeling excited, not wanting to sleep, having lots of energy coupled with a strong libidinal drive are all typical features that most adolescents will experience regularly from time to time. Hence, a diagnosis of bipolar II may not be made even though several episodes of hypomania may well have occurred. However, even if a diagnosis of bipolar II disorder is assigned, having determined that hypomanic episodes have occurred, this is not fixed, as it may be supplanted by a full-blown manic syndrome. Thus, a mood disorder diagnosis can undergo stepwise changes that eventuate in significant changes overall, which can have major implications for illness course, treatment, and prognosis.

Therefore, a longitudinal perspective is critical, and it is the assessment of functioning and likely impairment that is subtly imbedded within the criteria for each episode that is critical for meaningful appraisal. Here again, the lack of specific cut-offs means that these evaluations depend on clinical judgement, and for the time being at least, this latitude is probably for the best.

References

1. World Health Organization. (2018). *International Statistical Classification of Diseases and Related Health Problems* (11th revision). Geneva: World Health Organization.
2. Angst, J., Ajdacic-Gross, V., Rössler, W. (2020). Bipolar disorders in ICD-11: current status and strengths. *Intl J Bipolar Disord*, 8(1), 3.
3. Malhi, G.S., Bell, E. (2022). Questions in psychiatry (QuiP): sexual well-being and mental illness. *Bipolar Disord*, 24(1), 86–89. https://doi.org/10.1111/bdi.13179
4. Malhi, G.S., Irwin, L., Hamilton, A., et al. (2018). Modelling mood disorders: an ACE solution? *Bipolar Disord*, 20, 4–16.
5. Bell, E., Boyce, P., Porter, R.J., Bryant, R. A., Malhi, G.S. (2021). Irritability in mood disorders: neurobiological underpinnings and implications for pharmacological intervention. *CNS Drugs*, 35(6), 619–641.

6. American Psychiatric Association. (2013). *Diagnostic and Statistical Manual of Mental Disorders: DSM-5*, 5th ed. Arlington, VA: American Psychiatric Publishing.
7. Mulder, R.T., Horwood, J., Tyrer, P., Carter, J., Joyce, P.R. (2016). Validating the proposed ICD-11 domains. *Personal Ment Health*, 10(2), 84–95.
8. Salk, R.H., Hyde, J.S., Abramson, L.Y. (2017). Gender differences in depression in representative national samples: meta-analyses of diagnoses and symptoms. *Psychol Bull*, 143(8), 783.
9. Duffy, A., Carlson, G., Dubicka, B., Hillegers, M.H.J. (2020). Pre-pubertal bipolar disorder: origins and current status of the controversy. *Intl J Bipolar Disord*, 8(1), 18.
10. Malhi, G.S., Bell, E., Hamilton, A., Morris, G. (2020). Paediatric Bipolar Disorder: prepubertal or premature? *Aust N Z J Psychiatry*, 54(5), 547–50.
11. Malhi, G.S., Bell, E. (2021). Questions in psychiatry (QuiP): is paediatric bipolar disorder a valid diagnosis? *Bipolar Disord*, 23(3), 297–300.
12. Parker, G. (2021). Polarised views: a critique of the mood disorders guidelines. *Aust N Z J Psychiatry*, 55(6).
13. Malhi, G.S. (2021). Thing one and thing two: what 'Doctors use' to doctor you? *Aust N Z J Psychiatry*, 55(6), 536–547.
14. Malhi, G.S., Fritz, K., Allwang, C., et al. (2015). Agitation for recognition by DSM-5 mixed features specifier signals fatigue? *Aust N Z J Psychiatry*, 49(6), 499–501.
15. Malhi, G.S., Bell, E., Bassett, D., et al. (2021). The 2020 Royal Australian and New Zealand College of Psychiatrists clinical practice guidelines for mood disorders. *Aust N Z J Psychiatry*, 55(1), 7–117.
16. Dunner, D.L. (2017). Bipolar II Disorder. *Bipolar Disord*, 19(7), 520–521.
17. Robins, E.L.I., Guze, S.B. (1970). Establishment of diagnostic validity in psychiatric illness: its application to schizophrenia. *Am J Psychiatry*, 126(7), 983–987.
18. Luty, J. (2020). Bordering on the bipolar: a review of criteria for ICD-11 and DSM-5 persistent mood disorders. *BJPsych Advances*, 26(1), 50–57.
19. Kraepelin, E. (1899). *Psychiatrie: ein Lehrbuch für Studirende und Aerzte* (Psychiatry: A Manual for Students and Physicians), 6th ed. Leipzig: Johann Ambrosius Barth.
20. Salvatore, P., Baldessarini, R.J., Centorrino, F., et al. (2002). Weygandt's On the Mixed States of Manic-Depressive Insanity: a translation and commentary on its significance in the evolution of the concept of bipolar disorder. *Harv Rev Psychiatry*, 10(5), 255–275.
21. Bell, E., Malhi, G.S., Mannie, Z., et al. (2021). Novel insights into irritability: the relationship between subjective experience, age and mood. *BJPsych Open*, 7(6), e198.
22. Mulder, R., Tyrer, P. (2019). Diagnosis and classification of personality disorders: novel approaches. *Curr Opin Psychiatry*, 32(1).
23. Tyrer, P., Mulder,öR., Kim, Y.-R., Crawford, M.J. (2019). The development of the ICD-11 Classification of Personality Disorders: an amalgam of science, pragmatism, and politics. *Ann Rev Clin Psychol*, 15(1), 481–502.
24. Bassett, D. (2012). Borderline personality disorder and bipolar affective disorder. Spectra or spectre? A review. *Aust N Z J Psychiatry*, 46(4), 327–339.
25. Singh, M.K., Chang, K.D., Goldstein, B.I., et al. (2020). Isn't the evidence base for pediatric bipolar disorder already sufficient to inform clinical practice? *Bipolar Disord*, 22(7), 664–665.
26. Malhi GS, Bell E. Fake views: DMDD, indeed! Australian and New Zealand Journal of Psychiatry. 2019;53(7):706–10.
27. Malhi, G.S., Bell, E. (2019). Fake views: DMDD, indeed! *Aust N Z J Psychiatry*, 53(7), 706–710.

Bipolar 'Hoo' Disorder

Gin S. Malhi

Response to Allen Frances

I was heartened to read in his first sentence on the matter that Allen Frances *'regret[s] adding Bipolar II to DSM-IV'*, as I wholeheartedly share his concern that *'it may be similarly misused'* within ICD-11. And this is precisely why I have been questioning the validity of the diagnosis for over a decade. If ever there was a case of *not* learning from one's mistakes, the story of Bipolar II disorder is a prime example. And if Allen, the chair of DSM-IV, belatedly repents his decision to include Bipolar II, perhaps we should also consider the sentiments of David Dunner, one of the architects of Bipolar II.

In his 2017 editorial[1] published in *Bipolar Disorders*, David points out that the duration of hypomania was initially proposed as 3 days or longer, and that this was based on his observations of *'healthy female medical students'* while conducting research as a resident. He goes on to clarify that 3 days was chosen as the cut-off because *'many of them described premenstrual episodes of elevated mood, but these never lasted longer than 2 days'*. This is an extraordinary revelation. But perhaps equally remarkable is his statement regarding the criteria used to define bipolar II as a separate diagnostic group in DSM-IV. Regarding this, he acknowledges that many of the purported *'differences supporting the separation of bipolar II as a distinct group have not been replicated'*. However, he rationalizes this failure, arguing that this is *'largely because there have been no attempts'*. I disagree. Over the past 40 years, plenty of attempts have been made using all manner of technologies, and many clinical indicators and so-called biomarkers have been proposed. But none has been corroborated, and overall, no substantive evidence has been found to reliably differentiate bipolar II disorder from its better-defined bedfellow.

In this same article, David also states that the *'the decision regarding the minimal duration of hypomania was set at 4 days or longer, and this decision was not based on data but rather on a concern of the leadership of DSM-IV to limit the diagnosis of bipolar II'*. In other words, the risks that Allen alludes to were clearly foreseen. David adds that subsequent DSM-5 adoptions of *'short duration (2–3 days) hypomania symptoms with major depressive episodes, and hypomania with insufficient symptoms with major depressive episodes'* are also *'not data based'*, and he concludes wistfully with a *'wish that these changes had been data based'*.

In retrospect, the DSM inclusion of Bipolar II disorder seems baffling, but perhaps even more puzzling is the fact that a diagnosis created on such arbitrary grounds persists to this day and continues to enjoy illness status. But even if we put the diagnostic concerns aside, the problem that is perhaps of greater concern is that the label lacks any meaningful implications for treatment.[2] And while Allen is correct in that *'patients with bipolar II pattern of symptoms* [also] *sort with Bipolar Disorder* [meaning bipolar I disorder]', surely this is to be expected given that it is after all the *same* illness?

Thus, to be clear, in my view, Bipolar II disorder lacks clinical distinction and has no neuroscientific foundation.[3] Its adoption by ICD-11 is an unfathomable mistake that has ensured the diagnosis will continue to be misused, and that the mistakes of the past will be repeated.

References

1. Dunner, D.L. (2017). Bipolar II disorder. *Bipolar Disord*, **19**(7), 520–521. https://doi.org/10.1111/bdi.12567
2. Malhi, G.S. (2021). Thing one and thing two: what 'doctors use' to doctor you? *Aust N Z J Psychiatry*, **55**(6), 536–547. https://doi.org/10.1177/00048674211022602
3. Malhi, G., Outhred, T., Irwin, L. (2019). Bipolar II Disorder is a myth. *Can J Psychiatry*, **64**(8), 531–536. https://doi.org/10.1177/0706743719847341

Chapter 5: Disorders Specifically Associated with Stress

Chris R. Brewin & Andreas Maercker

Post-Traumatic Stress Disorder (PTSD)

Essential and Associated Features

Post-traumatic stress disorder (PTSD) follows an event or situation that in the judgement of the clinician has been experienced by the individual as extremely threatening or horrific. Such events are not limited to those generally regarded as traumatic but may, if the result is that the person comes to experience extreme fear or horror, include experiences such as being repeatedly stalked, bullied, rejected, or humiliated.[1] Experiencing threatening delusions and hallucinations, and the atypical processing of the social and sensory world associated with conditions such as Autism Spectrum Disorder, may result in other types of experiences qualifying because they are subjectively experienced with extreme fear or horror.[2]

A PTSD diagnosis also requires the simultaneous presence of three core elements. The first element is evidence that the traumatic event is being re-experienced in the present. That is, the individual has the experience that the traumatic event is happening again in the 'here and now'. The re-experiencing may occur either in the form of nightmares that closely recapitulate the themes of the event (without necessarily reproducing it exactly), or in the form of daytime intrusive memories and flashbacks. The second core element is evidence of deliberate avoidance of the traumatic event, either in the form of internal avoidance of thoughts and memories, or of external avoidance of people, conversations, activities, or situations reminiscent of the event. The third core element is evidence of persistent perceptions of heightened current threat, for example as indicated by hypervigilance or by an enhanced startle reaction to stimuli such as unexpected noises. At least one symptom corresponding to each element must last for at least several weeks. Symptoms must also be accompanied by significant impairment in personal, family, social, educational, occupational, or other important areas of functioning.

Many other symptoms (e.g., irritability, sleep problems, impaired concentration) will commonly be encountered but are not unique to PTSD; they may indicate a co-occurring condition. Although fear and horror will be present to some degree, other emotions such as anger, shame, or guilt are often more prominent.

Parts of this chapter were prepared for a version of the chapter five years ago together with Heide Glaesmer and Richard A. Bryant.

Relation to Normality and Other Disorders

Most people who experience extremely threatening or horrific events do not develop a disorder. They may exhibit PTSD symptoms, but these are likely to subside quickly. If symptoms persist after a stressor that did not produce extreme fear or horror, other diagnoses should be considered. Depression, for example, is often accompanied by intrusive memories, but these are not usually re-experienced in the present. If the requirements for other disorders are not met, a diagnosis of Adjustment Disorder can be assigned. A variety of dissociative symptoms can occur following exposure to an extremely threatening or horrific event, including somatic symptoms and trance or fugue states, and a Dissociative Disorder may be considered as an alternative or co-occurring diagnosis if these symptoms are prominent. Both PTSD and Prolonged Grief Disorder may occur in individuals who experience bereavement as a result of the death of a loved one under traumatic circumstances. Unlike in PTSD, in which the individual re-experiences the event or situation associated with the death, in Prolonged Grief Disorder the person may be preoccupied with memories of the circumstances surrounding the death but does not re-experience them as occurring again in the here and now.

The disorders that most commonly co-occur with PTSD are Depressive Disorders, Anxiety or Fear-Related Disorders, and Disorders Due to Substance Use. Rates of comorbidity are very high, particularly with depression. Studies investigating the correlates of different latent factors of PTSD have found that symptoms characteristic of anxiety and depression appear to be more strongly related to those factors reflecting general dysphoria rather than to the more specific aspects of PTSD reflecting re-experiencing, active avoidance, and hyperarousal.[3]

Relation to ICD-10 and DSM-5

PTSD in ICD-10 had a similar focus on re-experiencing symptoms, but was a less specific disorder and did not require evidence of impairment. There were concerns about whether its high prevalence was realistic, and prevalence is reduced in ICD-11.[3] A DSM-5 diagnosis has a narrower definition of trauma exposure and requires the presence of four types of symptom, with a minimum of 6 out of 20 symptoms. Whereas ICD-11 focuses on those symptoms that distinguish PTSD from other disorders, DSM-5 seeks to provide a more comprehensive account of those symptoms that are commonly encountered, even though many are shared with other disorders. The prevalence of PTSD as measured by ICD-11 is usually slightly lower than when it is measured using DSM-5.[3]

The DSM-5 diagnosis of PTSD can be based on over half a million different combinations of symptoms,[4] which reduces its utility for scientific research. In contrast, ICD-11 PTSD can be assessed using as few as two symptoms per core element,[5] such that only 27 combinations of symptoms yield a diagnosis. It is hoped that in addition the greater specificity of ICD-11 PTSD will lead to it being recognized and treated more easily.

Complex PTSD

Essential and Associated Features

In Complex PTSD (CPTSD), all diagnostic requirements for PTSD are met. In addition, CPTSD is characterized by three additional core elements describing disturbances in self-organization, all of which must be present.[6] The first element is severe and persistent problems in affect regulation. This can be reflected in hyper-reactivity, for example difficulty recovering from minor stressors, having violent outbursts, or behaving recklessly, or in hypo-reactivity, for example emotional numbing, difficulty experiencing pleasure or positive emotions (anhedonia), and dissociation (e.g., feeling outside of one's body, feeling the world is unreal, gaps in memory). The second element consists of pervasive and persistent beliefs about oneself as being diminished, defeated, or worthless, accompanied by feelings of shame, guilt, or failure related to the traumatic event. The third element involves persistent and pervasive difficulties in sustaining relationships and in feeling close to others, as reflected, for example, in avoidance of relationships, ending relationships when difficulties or conflicts emerge, or deriding the value or importance of relationships. These symptoms cause significant impairment in personal, family, social, educational, occupational, or other important areas of functioning.

Although CPTSD is a disorder that most commonly develops following prolonged or repetitive events from which escape is difficult or impossible (e.g., torture, domestic violence, repeated childhood sexual or physical abuse), chronic trauma is a risk factor, not a requirement, for the diagnosis of Complex PTSD. Thus, CPTSD may be diagnosed following a single traumatic event, and PTSD following chronic or prolonged trauma. This approach recognizes the importance of multiple risk and resilience factors arising from personal attributes, environmental resources, and biological variables.

Associated features of CPTSD include suicidal ideation or behaviour and substance abuse, which may be related to emotion regulation difficulties. There is a substantial subgroup with psychotic symptoms.[7] Somatic complaints may be present but can also be a more direct result of the traumatic events themselves. Pervasive dissociation may be present, including fugue states and a complete loss of awareness of the current environment occurring in therapy sessions and in everyday situations such as crossing roads.

Response to Criticism of Allen Frances

Allen Frances (in Chapter 2 of this book) suggests that ICD-11 Complex PTSD is simply a severe form of ICD-11 PTSD. This has been tested using factor mixture modelling, a technique that combines dimensional (factor analysis) and categorical (mixture modelling) analysis. Two recent studies have confirmed that ICD-11 PTSD and Complex PTSD form distinct latent classes and do not simply differ on a severity dimension. The term 'Complex PTSD' is also popular and found to be useful by clinicians. In ICD-11, it has a number of features that clearly demarcate from earlier versions, including being easier to define and measure. There is every reason to think that over time the ICD-11 version of Complex PTSD will come to be preferred to previous versions, bringing with it important advantages in diagnostic specificity.

Relation to Normality and Other Disorders

Personality Disorders are also typified by pervasive problems in functioning related to the self and interactions with others. They differ in that the presence of the symptoms must have persisted over an extended period (generally 2 years or more) and is not specifically tied to a traumatic stressor. Symptom duration may be shorter in Complex PTSD, which also, unlike Personality Disorders, requires the presence of a traumatic stressor and consequent PTSD symptoms.

A diagnosis of Personality Disorder can include a qualifier for 'borderline pattern'. This pattern describes similar domains of disturbance to Complex PTSD but the nature of the problems is different and the two conditions can be discriminated empirically.[8,9] In the Borderline pattern, self-concept difficulties reflect an instability in identity with shifting overly positive or overly negative self-appraisals, whereas in Complex PTSD the self-concept is stable but persistently negative. Relational difficulties in the context of the Borderline Pattern are characterized by volatile patterns of interactions with alternating over-idealization or denigration of the other person, whereas in Complex PTSD relational difficulties are characterized by a persistent tendency to avoid relationships and distancing in times of difficulties.

Following an experience of a traumatic event, individuals with Complex PTSD may experience a variety of dissociative symptoms including somatic symptoms and trance or fugue state. These symptoms are also experienced by individuals with PTSD but are more strongly associated with and occur at substantially higher levels of severity among those with Complex PTSD.[10] The presence of persistent experiences of a fugue or trance state may warrant an additional diagnosis of Dissociative Disorder diagnosis.

Relation to ICD-10 and DSM-5

The ICD-10 included the condition 'Enduring personality change after catastrophic experience' (EPCACE) that also described disturbances in self-organization that can sometimes result from multiple, chronic, or repeated traumatic events. In contrast to EPCACE, CPTSD does not require exposure to chronic trauma or a demonstrable personality change, but it does require the presence of more specific symptoms, including PTSD symptoms. There is preliminary evidence that CPTSD is more readily distinguished by clinicians than EPCACE.[11] DSM-5 does not recognize CPTSD. Alternative formulations of Complex PTSD such as Disorders of Extreme Stress Not Otherwise Specified (DESNOS) have been considered by the DSM-IV and DSM-5 but insufficient evidence was found to support them. DSM-5 PTSD includes a number of the symptoms of ICD-11 CPTSD.

Prolonged Grief Disorder

Essential and Associated Features

Prolonged Grief Disorder (PGD) describes a disturbance in which, following the death of a person close to the bereaved, there is persistent and pervasive yearning or longing for the deceased, or a persistent preoccupation with the deceased. Yearning and longing are the unbidden, repetitive desires for a cherished person from the past, often using imagery to conjure the deceased in the present.[12] These symptoms extend beyond 6 months after the loss, and the disorder is sufficiently severe to cause significant impairment in the person's functioning. Importantly, the disturbance goes far beyond expected social or cultural norms and depends on cultural and contextual factors.

The associated features are related to the preoccupation with the deceased or with the circumstances of the death, which may sometimes oscillate between preoccupation and avoidance of reminders. Intense emotional pain in PGD is often manifested by bitterness about the loss, sadness, guilt, anger, denial, or blame. Persons with PGD often have difficulty accepting the death and feel as if they have lost a part of themselves. Specific other symptoms may be apparent, for example an inability to experience positive mood, emotional numbness and difficulty experiencing feelings, or the feeling that life is meaningless. PGD has been associated with marked occupational and social impairment[13] that may be expressed, for example, by difficulty progressing with activities, or by withdrawal, or difficulty in engaging with social or other activities.

Relation to Normality and Other Disorders

An individual who experiences a grief reaction that is within a normative period in their cultural and religious context is considered a normal griever and should not be given a diagnosis of prolonged grief disorder. Thereafter, it is the intensity of the grief symptoms and whether they significantly impair the person's life that determine whether this diagnosis should be assigned. In this context, it is important to take into account whether other people who share the grieving person's cultural or religious mindset (e.g., family, friends, community) may view the reaction to the loss or the duration of the reaction as abnormal. Therefore, cultural considerations about the person's frame of reference and the normative length of the grieving phase in the respective culture are key.[14]

Response to Allen Frances

Allen Frances' criticism can be countered. He states in Chapter 2 that 'there can never be a uniform expiration date on normal grief – and ICD-11 should not have felt empowered to impose one. People grieve in their own ways, for periods of time that vary widely depending on the person; the nature of the loss; and relevant cultural practices.' In the ICD-11 revision, we recognized that time definitions are not ideal in coding psychopathology. We have therefore chosen soft definitions such as 'usually/at least etc.' For PGD, it has been emphasized that the time criterion – approximately 6 months – can be varied according to the cultural circumstances of the reference population. Accordingly, the European or Christian (actually Catholic) 'year of mourning' can be varied in national versions of ICD-11, for example, in the US or German-language versions. The time criterion 'approximately 6 months' was established after intensive best-practice-based discussions, especially by the non-Western representatives (Asia, Africa, South America) of the working group. In China, Japan, and Korea, by the way, the new diagnosis was unanimously strongly welcomed and seen as a missing component of psychopathology. There are over two dozen publications on it from these countries.

Frances also claims in Chapter 2, 'Mislabelling grief as mental disorder stigmatizes the grievers; exposes them to unneeded psychiatric medication; and insults the dignity of their loss.' ICD-11 has been developed with psychiatrists, clinical psychologists, social workers, and psychiatric nurses. Therefore, it is quite wrong to assume prescribing medication automatically to the patients in question. Many professional groups would be very reluctant to prescribe. Loss of dignity on this diagnosis would be strongly denied by our Asian colleagues. On the contrary: they think that globally many of the conditions automatically diagnosed as full-scale depressive disorders might actually be grief sequelae conditions and so reduce drug prescribing.

The two main diagnoses that can overlap with PGD are PTSD and depression. Whereas both PGD and PTSD can involve intrusive memories of the deceased, PTSD memories tend to be focused on fearful events that trigger marked avoidance; in contrast, PGD can also involve intrusive memories of the deceased, but these typically evoke sadness and the person can also have positive memories of the deceased. Whereas both depression and PGD involve dysphoric mood, depression is marked by a constant dysphoric mood state; PGD, on the other hand, involves sadness that is typically elicited by reminders of the loss.[15]

Relation to ICD-10 and DSM-5

The diagnosis Prolonged Grief Disorder was not available in ICD-10. As a result, people with the condition were usually given an imprecisely formulated diagnosis of depression or, in a few cases, were diagnosed with adjustment disorder. In ICD-11, PGD can be seen as a sister diagnosis of adjustment disorder.

In the original version of the DSM-5, published in 2013, no diagnosis of persistent grief disorder was included, but a proposed diagnosis was added to the Appendix in recognition that the construct required further research (termed Persistent Complex Bereavement Disorder). The editorial revision of the DSM-5 in 2020 included PGD as a new diagnosis.[16] Its criteria largely overlap with those in ICD-11 insofar as they place core emphasis on yearning and preoccupation for the deceased with associated indicators of disruption. It departs from the ICD-11 definition in some key ways. The DSM-5 criteria require the person to have persistent yearning for at least 12 months after the death (6 months for children), and at least three of a possible eight symptoms that extend beyond those outlined in ICD-11: these include emotional numbness and intense loneliness.

Adjustment Disorder

Essential and Associated Features

Adjustment disorder (AjD) is a maladaptive reaction to identifiable psychosocial stressors or life changes characterized by the two symptom groups of preoccupation with the stressor and failure to adapt. Preoccupation with the stressor can be defined as stressor-related factual thinking, which is time-consuming and associated with negative emotions.[17] Failure to adapt may be manifested by a range of symptoms that interfere with everyday functioning, such as difficulties concentrating or sleeping. The symptoms emerge within a month of the onset of the stressor or stressors and tend to resolve in 6 months unless the stressor persists for a longer duration. In order to be diagnosed, adjustment disorder must be associated with significant distress and significant impairment in personal, family, social, educational, occupational, or other important areas of functioning.

Associated features consist of symptoms of depression (e.g., depressed mood, hopelessness), anxiety (e.g., a state of anxiety when thinking about the stressful situation), and impulsivity (e.g., quickly losing temper, feeling restless and nervous), and are conceptualized as associated features of AjD.

Relation to Normality and Other Disorders

First, AjD must be distinguished from normal stress responses. Then it must be differentiated from other mental disorders such as mood disorders and anxiety disorders. This can be challenging since there is symptom overlap between AjD and these conditions. The symptoms may represent a depressive episode in evolution. However, in AjD the onset of symptoms is clearly related to a stressor and the presence of a stressor is essential to making the diagnosis. In contrast, anxiety and depressive disorders can develop without any stressor but some stressful event is frequently reported. In these, a stressor is not essential. Moreover, symptoms of depression and anxiety in AjD may also be less severe. It is important to also recognize that not everybody who experiences a traumatic event develops PTSD and, if the full criteria are not met, AjD may be a more appropriate diagnosis. In addition, AjD has to be distinguished from Prolonged Grief Disorder, which is characterized by a pattern of yearning or longing symptoms for the deceased or by a persistent preoccupation with the circumstances of the death.

Response to Allen Frances

In Chapter 2, Allen Frances argues that adjustment disorder could be used frequently instead of PGD and advises practitioners not to 'follow any ICD-11-induced fad to suddenly pathologize what is one of humanity's most ubiquitous, basic, and essential life experiences'.

In responding to this, we are not indifferent to possible overlap with other conditions. Our colleague Richard Bryant, from Australia, has argued the case for PGD cogently:

> There has been accumulating evidence over many years validating prolonged grief disorder as a specific and identifiable condition that can severely impact a minority of bereaved people. There are many factor-analytic studies indicating that the construct of persistent yearning and emotional pain, together with its associated symptoms, is a well-defined syndrome, and that this syndrome is distinct from other related disorders such as depression and adjustment disorder.[18]

There is a great deal more information from worldwide studies that cannot be included in this chapter due to lack of space.

Relation to ICD-10 and DSM-5

The ICD-10 definition of AjD was often criticized because it did not include positive diagnostic criteria, as is now the case with the symptoms of preoccupation and failure to adapt. It was a diagnosis of exclusion only, which made it a 'wild card' in the diagnostic process, albeit unsatisfactory for scientific and public health reasons.[19] For example, in some countries such as the Netherlands the ICD-10 AjD diagnosis was no longer sufficient to be used for health insurance or social welfare legislation. The introduction of the ICD-11 AjD diagnosis was not accompanied by increased AjD prevalence rates compared to ICD-10, instead the rates appear comparable in population studies.[20]

There are commonalities between the diagnostic criteria for AjD in DSM-5 and ICD-11 in terms of the presence of a stressor in close temporal relationship to the onset of symptoms. Beyond that, there are few similarities. The time from the stressor to the onset of symptoms is different; DSM-5 requires symptoms or impairment, whereas ICD-11 requires both. The criteria in DSM-5 are very broad, in contrast to ICD-11 where they are much more specific. DSM-5 retains the subtypes, while ICD-11 does not. Finally, DSM-5 still regards AjD as a disorder without positive symptom specification and thus, unlike ICD-11, as a subthreshold disorder. These differences are likely to lead to research developments that may diverge from the approach of DSM-5, particularly in terms of the introduction of a more distinct characterization of the core features of AjD and its elevation to full threshold status.

Reactive Attachment Disorder and Disinhibited Social Engagement Disorder

The ICD-11 includes two disorders unique to childhood with onset ages between 1 and 5 years, both arising from a history of grossly insufficient care. The degree of deprivation implies that these disorders may often be accompanied by a more global impact on cognition (e.g., working memory deficits), behaviour (e.g., temper tantrums), and affective functioning (e.g., difficulty regulating emotions). Although defined as disorders of early childhood, there is growing interest in the extent to which the same symptoms may be manifest in school-age children and adolescents, particularly those with a history of institutional care.[21,22] At this later age, the disorders are also likely to be comorbid with other psychiatric disorders and psychosocial problems.[23]

The requirement for Reactive Attachment Disorder (RAD) in ICD-11 is a pattern of emotionally withdrawn behaviour towards more than one caregiver, shown by minimal comfort-seeking and minimal response to comfort when offered. In ICD-10, RAD was characterized more broadly in terms of persistent abnormalities in social relationships, which could include fearfulness and hypervigilance, poor social interaction with peers, aggression towards self and others, misery, and growth failure. In DSM-5, RAD is described as a chronic pattern of being emotionally withdrawn and inhibited, which is demonstrated by rarely seeking or being responsive to comfort when distressed. Moreover, there is other evidence of emotional disturbance such as episodes of irritability, fearfulness, or sadness that are out of proportion to the situation.

The requirement for Disinhibited Social Engagement Disorder in ICD-11 is a lack of reticence with unfamiliar adults, shown by over-familiarity, lack of checking, and willingness to go off with them. This is similar to ICD-10, which mentioned diffuse, non-selectively focused attachment behaviour, attention-seeking, indiscriminately friendly behaviour, and poorly modulated peer interactions. Likewise, DSM-5 specifies a pattern of behaviour in which a child shows reduced or absent reticence in approaching and interacting with unfamiliar adults, overly familiar verbal or physical behaviour, diminished or absent checking back with adult caregiver after venturing away, and willingness to go off with an unfamiliar adult with minimal or no hesitation.

Other Specified Disorders Specifically Associated with Stress

This category may be used for individuals exposed to stress or trauma who present with symptoms similar to other Disorders Specifically Associated with Stress, but do not fulfil the diagnostic requirements for any of them. The diagnosis requires that the symptoms are not better accounted for by another mental disorder such as anxiety disorder or depression, and that they are accompanied by significant distress or functional impairment.

General Discussion

The changes made in ICD-11 reflect several decades of experience concerning the strengths and weaknesses of previous diagnoses subsumed under the category of stress and trauma-related disorders. The PTSD diagnosis, first introduced in 1980, has been extraordinarily successful in raising the profile of traumatic stress and changing the landscape of psychopathology and psychological intervention. Among its limitations are an evidence base heavily reliant on observations of groups such as domestic violence survivors and military veterans. Over the years, it has undergone several revisions to the way traumatic stressors are defined and to its constituent symptoms. Concerns have been raised about the complexity of the diagnosis and about its ability to adequately reflect the impact of experiences such as early childhood trauma. ICD-11 addresses both these concerns by simplifying the diagnosis and distinguishing PTSD and Complex PTSD.

These changes represent a very distinct alternative to the way PTSD is diagnosed using successive versions of the DSM. To date, there is substantial empirical evidence for the factorial validity of PTSD and Complex PTSD and for the distinction between them.[24,25] Most of the symptoms are familiar, but the narrowing of the focus on re-experiencing in the present rather than any kind of intrusive thought or memory may take some time to be fully appreciated.[11] Ultimately, the utility of this new approach awaits verification through everyday clinical practice. One important issue will be to determine who would have received a PTSD diagnosis under the DSM but not under ICD-11, and whether their symptoms are better captured by another disorder.

Evidence from community samples suggests that the number of children diagnosed with DSM-based PTSD is very similar to the number receiving either a PTSD or CPTSD diagnosis in ICD-11.[3] Despite this, the overlap in case identification is modest and more needs to be understood about which children receive a DSM but not an ICD-11 diagnosis, and vice versa.[26] Relatively little is known about the differences in functioning of the DSM-IV, DSM-5 pre-school, and ICD-11 criteria in samples of younger and preadolescent children.[27] Importantly, the distinction between PTSD and CPTSD appears to be equally valid in samples of children.[28,29]

With regard to PGD, the available evidence highlights the importance of having a specific diagnosis to identify people with persistent and severe grief reactions. Such a diagnosis can facilitate provision of optimal treatment for chronically distressed people after bereavement. Considering the number of people who are bereaved globally each year, it can be estimated that millions of people may suffer from PGD, and so it is important to be able to develop simple and accurate methods of identifying these individuals in order for strategies to be implemented to alleviate their potentially debilitating distress.

Adjustment disorder too has been changed from its ill-defined state to a thoroughly contemporary diagnosis based on basic psychological research and defined by positive criteria. Again, the utility of the proposals awaits clinical verification.

The advent of the new disorders specifically associated with stress under ICD-11 will require new measurement tools. To date, a number of questionnaires have been developed, including the International Trauma Questionnaire,[5] the International Prolonged Grief Disorder Scale,[30] the International Adjustment Disorder Questionnaire,[31] and the Adjustment Disorder New Module.[32] These are freely available from the website www.traumameasuresglobal.com. In the future, corresponding clinical interviews will be a matter of priority.

References

1. Hyland, P., Karatzias, T., Shevlin, M., et al. (2021). Does requiring trauma exposure affect rates of ICD-11 PTSD and Complex PTSD? Implications for DSM-5. *Psychol Trauma*, **13**(2), 133–141.
2. Brewin, C.R., Rumball, F., Happe, F. (2019). Neglected causes of post-traumatic stress disorder. *BMJ*, 365.
3. Brewin, C.R., Cloitre, M., Hyland, P., et al. (2017). A review of current evidence regarding the ICD-11 proposals for diagnosing PTSD and complex PTSD. *Clin Psychol Rev*, **58**, 1–15.
4. Galatzer-Levy, I.R., Bryant, R.A. (2013). 636,120 ways to have posttraumatic stress disorder. *Perspect Psychol Sci*, **8**(6), 651–662.
5. Cloitre, M., Shevlin, M., Brewin, C.R., et al. (2018). The International Trauma Questionnaire: development of a self-report measure of ICD-11 PTSD and complex PTSD. *Acta Psychiatr Scand*, **138**(6), 536–546.

6. Brewin, C.R. (2020). Complex posttraumatic stress disorder: a new diagnosis in ICD-11. *BJPsych Adv*, **25**(3), 145–152.

7. Frost, R., Vang, M.L., Karatzias, T., Hyland, P., Shevlin, M. (2019). The distribution of psychosis, ICD-11 PTSD and complex PTSD symptoms among a trauma-exposed UK general population sample. *Psychosis*, **11**(3), 187–198.

8. Hyland, P., Karatzias, T., Shevlin, M., Cloitre, M. (2019). Examining the discriminant validity of complex posttraumatic stress disorder and borderline personality disorder symptoms: results from a United Kingdom population sample. *J Trauma Stress*, **32**(6), 855–863.

9. Knefel, M., Tran, U.S., Lueger-Schuster, B. (2016). The association of posttraumatic stress disorder, complex posttraumatic stress disorder, and borderline personality disorder from a network analytical perspective. *J Anxiety Disord*, **43**, 70–78.

10. Hyland, P., Shevlin, M., Fyvie, C., Cloitre, M., Karatzias, T. (2020). The relationship between ICD-11 PTSD, complex PTSD and dissociative experiences. *J Trauma Dissociation*, **21**(1), 62–72.

11. Keeley, J.W., Reed, G.M., Roberts, M.C., et al. (2016). Disorders specifically associated with stress: a case-controlled field study for ICD-11 mental and behavioural disorders. *Int J Clin Health Psychol*, **16**, 109–127.

12. Robinaugh, D.J., Mauro, C., Bui, E., et al. (2016). Yearning and its measurement in complicated grief. *J Loss Trauma*, **21**(5), 410–420.

13. Boelen, P.A., Prigerson, H.G. (2007). The influence of symptoms of prolonged grief disorder, depression, and anxiety on quality of life among bereaved adults. *Eur Arch Psychiatry Clin Neurosci*, **257**(8), 444–452.

14. Killikelly, C., Maercker, A. (2017). Prolonged grief disorder for ICD-11: the primacy of clinical utility and international applicability. *Eur J Psychotraumatol*, **8**.

15. Shear, M.K. (2015). Complicated grief. *N Engl J Med*, **372**(2), 153–160.

16. Prigerson, H.G., Kakarala, S., Gang, J., Maciejewski, P.K. (2021). History and status of prolonged grief disorder as a psychiatric diagnosis. *Ann Rev Clin Psychol*, **17**, 109–126.

17. Eberle, D.J., Maercker, A. (2021). Preoccupation as psychopathological process and symptom in adjustment disorder: a scoping review. *Clin Psychol Psychother*, **29**(2), 455–468.

18. Tsai, W.I., Kuo, S.C., Wen, F.H., Prigerson, H.G., Tang, S.T. (2018). Prolonged grief disorder and depression are distinct for caregivers across their first bereavement year. *Psychooncology*, **27**(3), 1027–1034.

19. Bachem, R., Casey, P. (2018). Adjustment disorder: a diagnosis whose time has come. *J Affect Disord*, **227**, 243–253.

20. Glaesmer, H., Romppel, M., Braehler, E., Hinz, A., Maercker, A. (2015). Adjustment disorder as proposed for ICD-11: dimensionality and symptom differentiation. *Psychiatry Res*, **229**(3), 940–948.

21. Guyon-Harris, K.L., Humphreys, K.L., Degnan. K., et al. (2019). A prospective longitudinal study of Reactive Attachment Disorder following early institutional care: considering variable- and person-centered approaches. *Attach Hum Dev*, **21**(2), 95–110.

22. Seim, A.R., Jozefiak, T., Wichstrom, L., Kayed, N.S. (2020). Validity of reactive attachment disorder and disinhibited social engagement disorder in adolescence. *Eur Child Adolesc Psychiatry*, **29**(10), 1465–1476.

23. Seim, A.R., Jozefiak, T., Wichstrom. L., Lydersen, S., Kayed, N.S. (2022). Reactive attachment disorder and disinhibited social engagement disorder in adolescence: co-occurring psychopathology and psychosocial problems. *Eur Child Adolesc Psychiatry*, **31**(1), 85–98.

24. McElroy, E., Shevlin, M., Murphy, S., et al. (2019). ICD-11 PTSD and complex PTSD: structural validation using network analysis. *World Psychiatry*, **18**(2), 236–237.

25. Redican, E., Nolan, E., Hyland, P., et al. (2021). A systematic literature review of factor analytic and mixture models of ICD-11 PTSD and CPTSD using the International Trauma Questionnaire. *J Anxiety Disord*, **79**.

26. Danzi, B.A., La Greca, A.M. (2016). DSM-IV, DSM-5, and ICD-11: identifying children with posttraumatic stress disorder after disasters. *J Child Psychol Psychiatry*, **57**(12), 1444–1452.

27. Danzi, B.A., La Greca, A.M., Greif Green, J., Comer, J.S. (2021). What's in a name? Comparing alternative conceptualizations of posttraumatic stress disorder among preadolescent children following the Boston Marathon bombing and manhunt. *Anxiety Stress Coping*, **34**(5), 545–558.

28. Haselgrube, A., Solva, K., Lueger-Schuster, B. (2020). Validation of ICD-11 PTSD and complex PTSD in foster children using the International Trauma Questionnaire. *Acta Psychiat Scand*, **141**(1), 60–73.

29. Sachser, C., Keller, F., Goldbeck, L. (2017). Complex PTSD as proposed for ICD-11: validation of a new disorder in children and adolescents and their response to Trauma-Focused Cognitive Behavioral Therapy. *J Child Psychol Psychiatry*, **58**(2), 160–168.

30. Killikelly, C., Zhou, N., Merzhvynska, M., et al. (2020). Development of the international prolonged grief disorder scale for the ICD-11: measurement of core symptoms and culture items adapted for Chinese and German-speaking samples. *J Affect Disord*, **277**, 568–576.

31. Shevlin, M., Hyland, P., Ben-Ezra, M., et al. (2020). Measuring ICD-11 adjustment disorder: the development and initial validation of the International Adjustment Disorder Questionnaire. *Acta Psychiatr Scand*, **141**(3), 265–274.

32. Ben-Ezra, M., Mahat-Shamir, M., Lorenz, L., Lavenda, O., Maercker, A. (2018). Screening of adjustment disorder: Scale based on the ICD-11 and the Adjustment Disorder New Module. *J Psychiatric Res*, **103**, 91–106.

Chapter 6

Disorders Due to Substance Use

John B. Saunders

Introduction

Disorders due to substance use include some of the major causes of morbidity and mortality worldwide. Alcohol accounts for 3 million deaths worldwide and 5.1% of the global burden of disease and is the leading cause of premature mortality and disability among people aged 15–49 years, accounting for 10% of all deaths in this age group.[1] Tobacco, typically in the form of cigarettes, and with nicotine as the pharmacological addictive driver, is the cause of 8.7 million deaths and 7.9% of the global burden of disease.[2] Among the 25- to 49-year-old age group, psychoactive drug use causes 2.9% of the global burden of disease,[3] deaths having increased by 70% over the past decade, and opioids accounting for 70% of them.[4] Prescribed opioids and sedative-hypnotics also claim significant morbidity and mortality.

The World Health Organization, which has the responsibility of developing, reviewing, and updating the International Classification of Diseases (ICD), adopts a public health approach to substance use in supporting its strategic approach to minimizing overall harm.[5] In the 11th Revision of the ICD (ICD-11), which was approved by the World Health Assembly in May 2019[6] and was published in extended form for mental health disorders in 2021, substance use disorders are grouped with those due to addictive behaviours in a new section termed 'Disorders due to Substance Use and Addictive Behaviours'. The present chapter covers the 'Disorders due to Substance Use'[7] and also relevant substance-related health risk factors. A separate chapter in the ICD classification covers this subject.

The aims of the chapter are several:

1. to describe and comment upon the key diagnoses of substance use that feature in the ICD-11;
2. to provide a brief historical background for these diagnoses and the processes by which the ICD-11 diagnoses were generated and determined;
3. to compare the ICD-11 diagnoses with their nearest equivalent in ICD-10 – this will also include data analyses and field testing;
4. to compare the ICD-11 diagnoses with their nearest counterparts in the Fifth Edition of the *Diagnostic and Statistical Manual of Mental Disorders (DSM-5)*[8] which was published by the American Psychiatric Association in 2013.

There are several reasons for grouping the various disorders due to substance use. They include:

(1) The essential features of these disorders are typically shared among the substances that are included.[9] With limited exceptions, they have psychoactive properties, which at least initially are pleasurable. There are variations in disorders such as intoxication and withdrawal which reflect the differences in the pharmacological properties of

individual substances.[7] The 'limited exception' is that the section includes disorders due to non-psychoactive substances such as laxatives and growth hormone where these are taken repetitively and not for therapeutic purposes.
(2) These disorders have common genetic underpinnings and behavioural and neurobiological mechanisms.[10,11]
(3) These disorders have similar psychological antecedents, including the effects of adverse experiences such as abuse and trauma, and comorbidities.[12]
(4) There are similar sociocultural influences that affect the development and expression of these disorders. Correspondingly, however, sociocultural factors may explain differences[13] in how certain substances affect individuals and peoples from different cultures, examples including cocaine and kava.
(5) Similar assessment methods are used to gauge (i) the level of consumption, (ii) the presence of dependence (addiction), and (iii) physical and mental harm.[12]
(6) Similar approaches apply to the treatment of these disorders[12] including (i) psychological therapies, (ii) psychosocial supports, (iii) self- and mutual-help approaches, (iv) acceptance of personal responsibility, and (v) supportive environmental changes, which may include work, accommodation, domicile, and cultural understanding. The pharmacological treatments are often different between substance groups, reflecting their different pharmacological and neurobiological effects, but there are some medications used in common for the different disorders.

Background and Input to ICD-11

The predecessor to ICD-11, namely, the 10th revision, ICD-10, was published in 1992 in two forms. The first publication comprises brief descriptions of not only mental and behavioural disorders but all human conditions.[14] A subsequent publication was the *Clinical Descriptions and Diagnostic Guidelines* (the CDDG, or 'Blue Book'),[15] which covered mental and behavioural disorders (including those due to substance use) and was much expanded in content. It was intended to be equivalent in scope to its DSM counterpart. A third volume, the *Diagnostic Criteria for Research* (ICD-10 DCR),[16] was published in the following year. It was designed to complement the CDDG by providing more detailed and specific criteria, especially for characterizing participants in research studies including clinical trials. In the years since the publication of ICD-10, there have been many studies comparing its diagnostic utility compared with previous ICD revisions and also with Fourth Edition of the DSM (DSM-IV),[17] and as gauged by different diagnostic instruments.[18]

In the mid-2000s, the ICD-11 developmental process was initiated through a series of advisory groups and the production of discussion papers ('green papers'). In 2010, the Substance Use Disorders Workgroup was established. At its meetings, summaries of the relevant literature were presented and discussed. Draft descriptions and diagnostic guidelines of the major diagnoses expected to be included in ICD-11 were commissioned. Provisional diagnostic guidelines were presented at scientific meetings[19,20] and made available for public comment through the ICD-11 developmental platform on the WHO website. This was intended to ensure as full a consultation process as possible in a transparent way. A Global Clinical Practice Network exceeding 16,000 clinicians worldwide provided commentary on the proposed descriptions and guidelines.[21] This input was reviewed by the Alcohol, Drugs and Addictive Behaviour Unit of the Department of Mental Health and Substance Use, and the Classification and Terminologies Unit of WHO.

At an early stage, datasets which were of likely value for secondary data analyses were identified in a way similar to the DSM-5 process.[22,23] This subsequently led to secondary analyses of the ten-country World Mental Health Survey.[24] In addition, datasets from individual studies were analysed, where their question items could capture key substance use diagnoses in the ICD and DSM systems.[25] Concordance calculations were undertaken for the presumptive diagnoses in ICD-11 against their nearest equivalents in ICD-10, DSM-IV, and DSM-5. These datasets included both general population and clinical surveys.[26]

By early 2019, late-stage drafts of the brief definitions (ICD-11 for Mortality and Morbidity Statistics – ICD-11 MMS) and the ICD-11 CDDG for the Disorders due to Substance Use were available for further assessment. There followed a period of 18 months of field testing, largely undertaken through the global network of WHO collaborating centres. Feedback was provided by means of a structured questionnaire with free text sections which were collated by the collaborating centres, presented to a consensus conference, and then submitted to the WHO Headquarters.

As a result of all these inputs, amendments to some of the detail of the descriptions and in particular the subtypes and qualifiers were made. As an example, in the March 2019 draft CDDG, two time frames were specified for the diagnosis of Substance Dependence, namely, at least 12 months in general, but the diagnosis could be applied where 'use is continuous (daily or almost daily) for at least one month'. Input from the field-testing centres resulted in this second time period being revised to three months.

The Range of Substances

In ICD-11,[6,7] 14 substances/substance groups are specified and have distinct codes. This is an expansion from the nine that were listed in ICD-10.[14,15] Table 6.1 shows the substance groups in ICD-11 according to their primary pharmacological action.

The first task in establishing the diagnosis in ICD-11 is to identify the substance/substance group that predominates; the second is to determine the clinical syndrome (or syndromes) that applies. The reason for this order and focus on the substance in the ICD system is both for clinical and public health purposes. A vital task of health systems around the world and of WHO is to monitor the occurrence and prevalence of specific forms of

Table 6.1 Classification of substances by their pharmacological actions

CNS depressants	CNS stimulants	Other or mixed CNS actions
• Alcohol • Sedative-hypnotics and anxiolytics • Opioids • Volatile inhalants	• Nicotine • Cocaine • Stimulants (including amphetamine and methamphetamine) • Synthetic cathinones • Caffeine	• Cannabis • Synthetic cannabinoids • MDMA and related drugs • Hallucinogens • Dissociative drugs (e.g., ketamine and phencyclidine)

CNS, central nervous system.

substance use and their health impacts. These show considerable changes over time and differences from country to country. Understanding the pattern of substance use is important for health care systems nationally and globally.

In addition to these specified substances, there is provision in ICD-11 for the diagnosis of disorders due to 'Other specified psychoactive substances' and separately of disorders due to 'Non-psychoactive substances'.

The Hierarchy of Substance Use and Disorder

In human societies there is a spectrum of use of psychoactive substances.[27,28] This ranges for any particular person and substance from (1) zero use, (2) use which is low risk (e.g., low and infrequent episodes of alcohol consumption), (3) hazardous ('risky') use[27] where the level, frequency, or pattern of use is known from epidemiological or clinical studies to pose a risk of harmful consequences in the future, even though no evidence of harm presently exists, (4) single-episode use that has actually caused harm,[29] (5) a repeated pattern of use that has caused harm,[29] and (6) dependence when neurobiological changes have occurred leading to a persistent drive to continue using the substance[30] or 'addiction'. This hierarchy is depicted in Figure 6.1, which includes the four primary substance use diagnoses in ICD-11. One of the four primary diagnoses is expected to be made in every person who has a health problem related to substance use.

There is a specific purpose in emphasizing the spectrum of substance use and having four primary diagnoses in ICD-11 to capture those of clinical significance. The hierarchy reflects public health needs and approaches as enunciated by WHO and supports its core mission of minimizing harm and promoting health for all.

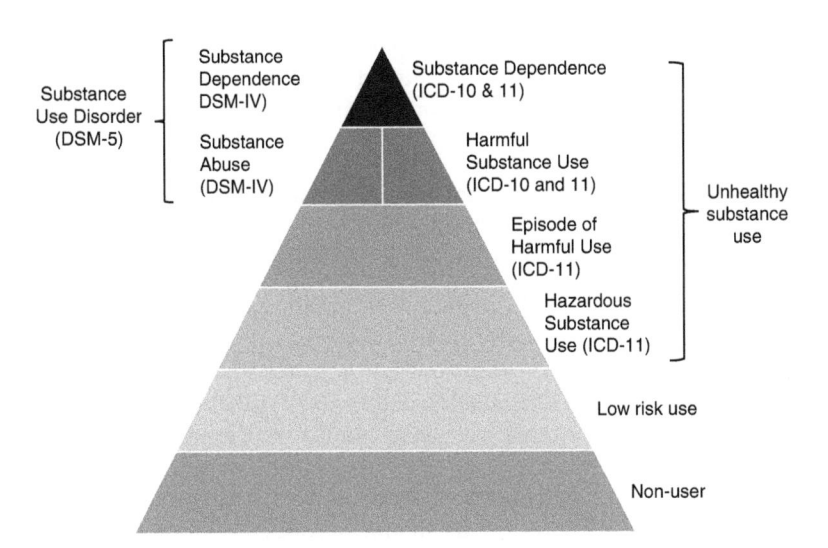

Figure 6.1 The Spectrum of Substance Use and Disorder, and the four Primary Substance Use Diagnoses.
1. There is a spectrum of substance use and disorder in human society.
2. This ranges for a particular substance from zero and low-risk use through hazardous (risky) use, use that has caused harm, to dependence on that substance.
3. This spectrum is illustrated in the 'pyramid' depicted here.
4. This informs the WHO public health approach.
5. The top four levels represent the primary substance use diagnoses, which are mutually exclusive.

Different policies, approaches, programmes, and models of service provision apply to each of the primary diagnoses.[5,31] Primary prevention is oriented in particular to those who are currently non-users or use at low-risk levels, with the aim of preventing uptake or escalation of use and reducing it with the aim of avoiding harmful consequences, now and in the longer term.[5] Screening and brief intervention apply particularly to those who are identified as having Hazardous Substance Use, and Harmful Substance Use (where the harm is not severe), with the aim of reducing use to lower-risk levels. Those diagnosed with Substance Dependence typically require fuller assessment and a detailed management plan, typically incorporating a programme of therapy, relapse-prevention, or agonist medications (as appropriate to the substance), and mutual help group involvement.[31] The goal of harm minimization is served by all these approaches, together with the strategy of harm reduction,[32,33] which aims to reduce substance-related harm despite the person continuing their existing pattern of substance use.

The Four Primary Diagnoses

The four primary diagnoses are set out below. As well as hierarchical, they are mutually exclusive, so only one can be diagnosed per substance (or substance group). However, different diagnoses may apply in the same individual to different substances (or substance groups).

Hazardous Substance Use

Hazardous Substance Use is a new diagnosis in ICD-11. It does not have a counterpart in ICD-10, although it was considered for inclusion and has been a WHO term since the 1980s.[27] It is a health risk factor, not a disorder. It is one of the primary diagnoses in ICD-11, at the lowest end of the spectrum but, importantly, signifying a pattern of substance use that confers a risk of harmful consequences. It is no longer included in ICD-11 but is part of a separate chapter entitled 'Disorders due to Substance Use and Addictive Behaviours'. This covers factors influencing health status or contact with health services. It is defined as:

> a pattern of substance use that is sufficient in frequency or quantity to increase appreciably the risk of harmful physical or mental health consequences to the user or to others to the extent that warrants attention and advice from health professionals.

The increased risk may arise from the frequency of substance use, from the amount used on a given occasion, from the cumulative total of substance use, or from risky behaviours associated with substance use or the context of use (e.g., use when operating machinery or electrical equipment), or from a combination of these. The risk may be related to the short-term effects of the substance or to longer-term cumulative effects on physical or mental health or functioning.

The diagnosis is best applied when there is epidemiological evidence linking a pattern or level of use to future harm, for example it would describe alcohol consumption of more than 100 grams of alcohol per week,[34] given that consumption above this amount is associated with a progressive increase in multiple physical and mental health consequences and increased all-cause mortality. It may be diagnosed when the clinician determines that a form of substance use is risky for that individual.

Harmful Substance Use

Harmful Substance Use is a diagnosis in ICD-10, which in ICD-11 is replaced by two separate diagnoses: 'Harmful Pattern of Substance Use' and 'Episode of Harmful Substance Use'.

Harmful Pattern of Substance Use

In ICD-11, this diagnosis is intended to capture a pattern of substance use which has led to harm, defined broadly as physical or mental, but in which the person does not fulfil the diagnostic guidelines for Substance Dependence. It corresponds therefore to the second dimension of the original bidimensional model of Edwards and colleagues[27,30] and which has had an enduring influence on nosological understanding. It may also be described as a sub-dependence diagnosis.

In ICD-11, it is defined as:

- a pattern of continuous, recurrent, or sporadic use of a psychoactive substance that has caused:
    - clinically significant damage to a person's physical ... or mental health ... or has resulted in behaviour leading to the harm of others.

Typically, the pattern is evident over 12 months or more. The second part of the definition represents an expansion over its ICD-10 counterpart in that the harm may be experienced by another person if it arises directly from the index individual's behaviour. Often, repeated intoxication would be the cause of the behaviour which leads to harm to others, but it may arise from behaviours independently of the intoxicated state.

The ICD-10 Harmful Substance Use did not have a direct counterpart in DSM-IV, with Substance Abuse in that system comprising social harm in the main. Likewise, the ICD-11 diagnosis does not relate closely to DSM-5 Substance Use Disorders.

Harm may occur to the individual because of 1) behaviour related to intoxication (e.g., aggressive behaviour, psychomotor impairment leading to injury), 2) direct or secondary toxic effects on body organs and systems (e.g., acute gastritis, chronic liver disease, exacerbation of pre-existing diseases), or 3) a harmful route of administration, for example injecting drug use. Where harm to the health of others has occurred, this may be manifested as any form of physical harm (e.g., trauma from substance-affected driving) or a mental disorder (e.g., post-traumatic stress disorder arising from an assault by the individual).

It is notable that many assessment questionnaires fail to capture physical or mental health problems arising from substance use, which has probably led to underdiagnosis of (ICD-10) Harmful Substance Use in studies reported in the scientific literature.

Episode of Harmful Substance Use

A new diagnosis in ICD-11 is 'Episode of Harmful Substance Use'. This was introduced to fill a gap in the classification where there was no diagnosis available to capture harm due to substance use (to the person or another) when there was no known pattern which would fulfil the guidelines for Harmful Substance Use or Substance Dependence. The diagnosis has particular application in emergency care or in other circumstances where detailed information on the history of substance use is not available, because the patient is too ill (e.g., unconscious) or is otherwise unable to give a detailed history and where collateral information is unavailable. Studies of patients presenting to emergency departments in 21 countries showed a prevalence of Episode of Harmful Alcohol Use in 16.3% of patients.[29]

As and when more information becomes available on any previous pattern of substance use, the diagnosis may be replaced by Harmful Pattern of Substance or Substance Dependence as appropriate.

Substance Dependence

At the top of the hierarchy is 'Substance Dependence'. This diagnosis featured in ICD-10[14,15] and DSM-IV,[35] and prior to this was included in the Third Edition, Revised (DSM-III-R).[36] It is the nearest equivalent in the ICD system to the old notions of addiction or 'alcoholism', but it is a much more specific concept than the older ones. In ICD-11[6] for the first time it has a conceptual definition as:

> A disorder of regulation of substance use that arises from repeated or continuous use of that substance and consists of a strong internal drive to use that substance.

The 'internal drive' is consequent on neurobiological changes[10,11] that develop as adaptive ones but become maladaptive and increasingly fixed.

The diagnosis requires a pattern of use that is manifested by two or more of the following key features:

- impaired control over substance use;
- increasing priority (or precedence) of substance use over other activities, such that substance use continues despite harm or negative consequences; and
- physiological features indicative of neuroadaptation to the substance, including (i) tolerance, (ii) withdrawal symptoms, or (iii) use to prevent or alleviate withdrawal.

The experiences are often accompanied by a subjective sensation of an urge ('craving') to use the substance, but this is not an obligatory feature. The description specifies a time frame of at least 12 months, but alternatively if use is continuous, the diagnosis may be made after 3 months.

The ICD-11 description and diagnostic guidelines of Substance Dependence represent a rationalization and a simplification of the corresponding ICD-10 diagnostic features.[15] Whereas this latter diagnosis required three or more of six essential features, the ICD-11 diagnosis has just three key features of which at least two need to be present. The rationale for this simplification is to promote understanding and utilization of these diagnoses, including importantly the communication that is facilitated between the clinician and the patient.

Such a rationalization needed to be empirically supported. Accordingly, during the developmental phase of ICD-11 secondary data analyses were undertaken to gauge the concordance of the proposed new diagnostic guidelines with those of ICD-10 and also with DSM-IV Substance Dependence. The concordance rates, as judged by the κ coefficient, were extremely high, averaging 0.95 for the diagnoses of Alcohol Dependence and Cannabis Dependence between the ICD-11 versions and those in ICD-10 and DSM-IV.[24,25]

The Components of Substance Dependence

Substance Dependence is a common diagnosis and most patients in a specialist facility who have a substance use disorder will have such a diagnosis. In considering whether a patient fulfils the guidelines for the diagnosis, the clinician should consider the context in which the three diagnostic guidelines may apply.

With regard to 'impaired control', this refers in the main to a typical episode of substance use. The clinician should seek to determine whether it had (i) exceeded the amount expected and resulted in intoxication or incapacity, (ii) extended beyond the time intended, (iii) resulted in the person experiencing difficulty in discontinuing use, (iv) occurred in inappropriate circumstances, or (v) was one of many recurring episodes.

By contrast, for 'increasing priority' a longitudinal perspective is necessary. The operative word is 'increasing'. This is not the same as 'greater' priority than something else at a single point in time. There should be evidence over time that the priority of substance use is increasing and is doing so to the extent that it is taking precedence over other aspects of life, other activities, and previous rewards and role responsibilities. In essence, the use of the substance takes 'centre stage' in that person's life and other activities and responsibilities are relegated to the periphery. Increasing priority is also evident when the person continues or increases their use of the substance in preference to maintaining their health and despite harmful consequences.

Physiological features, being the third key feature, are seen to a variable extent among the different substances. They contribute to the diagnosis but are not an obligatory requirement for it. This is because tolerance and particularly withdrawal do not appear to occur for certain substances, for example there is no recognized withdrawal state for hallucinogens. Also, physiological features are insufficient in themselves for the diagnosis of Substance Dependence. Where increased tolerance and withdrawal may be expected, for example in prescribing opioids for continuing cancer pain, the diagnosis of Substance Dependence should only be made if a key behavioural feature is also present, namely, 'impaired control' or 'increasing priority over other activities'. In this regard, prescription shopping ('doctor shopping') would be a pointer to increasing priority. This activity is uncommon in patients with cancer pain even though the doses of opioids may be extremely high, but it is much more common in patients who are taking prescription opioids for chronic non-malignant pain.

One of the diagnostic guidelines in ICD-10 Substance Dependence is 'craving', which was also introduced into DSM-5. This is a characteristic experience of many patients with Substance Dependence, but its occurrence varies from substance to substance, and it is affected by social desirability bias. It also tends to be difficult to translate into certain languages to convey the essence of what is a cognitive experience. Accordingly, it was excluded from the ICD-11 definition of Substance Dependence. Data analyses had shown that its deletion did not affect diagnostic concordance or prevalence, and earlier analyses in relation to DSM-5 showed that it neither contributed to nor detracted from the DSM-5 diagnosis of Substance Use Disorder.[37]

Substance Dependence and Harm

The diagnosis of ICD-11 Substance Dependence does not require that physical or mental harm should have occurred to the individual. In this regard the original bidimensional model[30] is maintained. Of course, physical and mental harm is very commonly seen in patients who fulfil the diagnosis of Substance Dependence, amounting to more than 90% of cases. With a diagnosis of ICD-11 Substance Dependence, specific forms of harm such as substance-induced mental disorders and substance-related physical disorders and injuries may be separately diagnosed, and this is encouraged for comprehensive diagnostic appraisal.

Comparisons with ICD-10 and DSM-5

As noted above, concordance of ICD-11 Substance Dependence with its ICD-10 counterpart is very high. In the World Mental Health Survey (WMHS), in which 8,841 individuals from 10 countries were interviewed, the concordance of ICD-11 Alcohol Dependence (three diagnostic guidelines) with its ICD-10 counterpart (six guidelines) was 0.95 (κ coefficient).[25] Concordance of ICD-11 Cannabis Dependence with its ICD-10 counterpart was 0.99.[25] High concordance rates were also seen for prescribed opioids.[26]

Concordance coefficients for the comparisons with DSM-IV diagnoses are similarly high. For Alcohol Dependence the κ coefficient was 0.99 and for Cannabis Dependence the κ value was 0.96.[25] (By contrast, the degree of diagnostic agreement with DSM-5 Substance Use Disorder is only moderate, hardly surprising given the broadening of the latter diagnosis from DSM-IV.) Even when the analyses were restricted to those with DSM-5 moderate/severe Alcohol Use Disorder, considered to be the nearest DSM diagnosis to ICD Alcohol Dependence, the κ value was only 0.63.[24] For the comparison with DSM-5 moderate/severe Cannabis Use Disorder, the κ value was 0.70.[25]

Prevalence comparisons, too, show broad agreement between the two ICD sets of diagnoses. The prevalence of ICD-11 Alcohol Dependence in the WMHS dataset was 6.8%, compared with 6.1% for ICD-10.[24] The results were widely disparate for the comparison with DSM-5 Alcohol Use Disorder (prevalence of 31.0%) and even for the moderate/severe subgroup (prevalence of 13.1%). The prevalence of ICD-11 Cannabis Dependence was 10.4%, compared with 10.2% for ICD-10, but was 28.1% for DSM-5 Cannabis Use Disorder and 15.9% for the moderate/severe subgroups.[24]

Consistent with most previous analyses for various substances of dependence, confirmatory factor analyses demonstrated that the ICD-11 alcohol and cannabis diagnoses were the best fit for a unifactorial model of substance dependence.

Additional Substance Use Diagnoses in ICD-11

Several additional diagnoses are available to capture particular clinical syndromes. These include Substance Intoxication (renamed from Acute Intoxication in ICD-10), Substance Withdrawal, and various substance-induced mental disorders.[6,7]

Substance Intoxication applies to all fourteen substance (groups) and specific features of Substance Intoxication are set out in ICD-11 for each one. Likewise, there are specific descriptions of Substance Withdrawal for each substance (group), with the exception of some such as hallucinogens where no identifiable withdrawal state has been described.

Four substance-induced mental disorders may be diagnosed for all fourteen substance (groups) and two additional ones are available specifically for various psychostimulants. These additional diagnoses may be made as required, in addition to one of the primary diagnoses.

In addition to these primary and additional diagnoses, further diagnoses of neurocognitive and psychomotor disorders may be made, as well as disorders of the sleep–wake cycle and disorders of sexual dysfunction. These other diagnoses have their primary location in other chapters of ICD-11, but a cross reference exists in the main chapter covering substance disorders. In addition, a range of physical disorders plus injuries may be diagnosed. Correspondingly, these diagnoses are found in those chapters in ICD-11 which deal with the respective organ or body system or injury.

Substance Intoxication

All the specified substances (Table 6.1) can result in states of intoxication. These range from mild but clinically relevant states to severe intoxication where the person's life may be seriously compromised. The features of substance intoxication reflect typically the primary pharmacological effects of the substance, namely, (i) CNS depressants, (ii) CNS stimulants, and (iii) substances with other or mixed effects. These include empathogens, hallucinogens, and dissociative drugs, and those with, for example, mixed stimulant and hallucinogenic properties (Table 6.1).

Substance Intoxication is defined in ICD-11 as the time-limited effects of high doses of psychoactive substances. It typically refers to discrete episodes of substance use; however, with repeated or continued use, the person may manifest features of intoxication for lengthy periods until that use ceases.

The generic definition of Substance Intoxication in ICD-11 is:

- transient and clinically significant disturbances in consciousness, cognition, perception, affect, behaviour, or coordination that develop during or shortly after consumption of a substance.

No specific features beyond these are found in the generic definition. Instead in the CDDG there are tables outlining the characteristic features of intoxication for each of the fourteen substances (groups).

Substance Intoxication is a clinical diagnosis. It may be supported by detection of the substance or a metabolite in urine, blood, or another body fluid, but the diagnosis should not be based merely on the presence or level of a substance. The features specified in the definition and the detailed descriptions must be present.

Substance Withdrawal

Substance Withdrawal also has a generic definition in ICD-11, namely, that it occurs in (some) persons with Substance Dependence (or who have prolonged and/or high-level substance use but may not have received that diagnosis) when they cease or reduce their level of use. Specific features of Substance Withdrawal depend on the pharmacological properties of the specified substance, and often they are the opposite of those acute effects, for example lethargy and inertia being characteristic features of stimulant withdrawal. The features should be consistent with those recognized as occurring upon cessation or reduction of that specific substance. The features vary in their nature, severity, and duration, and detailed descriptions of each withdrawal state are available. The diagnosis of Substance Withdrawal can be made when these features arise when prescribed psychoactive medications (e.g., opioids, anxiolytics, stimulants) have been taken, even when they have been used in standard therapeutic doses.

As mentioned above, Substance Withdrawal is one of the physiological features which can contribute to a diagnosis of Substance Dependence but does not automatically lead to that diagnosis.

Substance-Induced Mental Disorders

The ICD-11 provides for the diagnosis of various mental disorders which are considered to be induced by a psychoactive substance. These include:

- Substance-Induced Delirium;

- Substance-Induced Psychotic Disorder;
- Substance-Induced Mood Disorder; and
- Substance-Induced Anxiety Disorder.

These apply to all substances/substance groups. Two disorders apply only to psychostimulants, namely:

- Substance-Induced Obsessive–Compulsive Disorder; and
- Substance-Induced Impulse Control Disorder.

In addition, elsewhere in ICD-11 there are disorders of the sleep–wake cycle and disorders of sexual dysfunction, which may be diagnosed as substance induced.

Substance-induced mental disorders exist in a time frame between that of the short-term syndromes of Substance Intoxication and Substance Withdrawal, and the typically longer-term time frames of those mental disorders that have no direct aetiological relationship to substance use and are not clearly temporally related. Substance-induced mental disorders are diagnosed when there is a temporal relationship with substance use at or shortly after the onset of symptoms (and often during a state of intoxication or withdrawal) and where the features extend over several days, weeks, or occasionally months, beyond when a state of intoxication or withdrawal should have resolved. In contrast to DSM-5, where the criteria indicate that substance-induced mental disorders would normally be expected to resolve within or just after 1 month, ICD-11 specifies no exact duration. Most substance-induced mental disorders remit within several weeks, but some, for example alcohol- and stimulant-induced psychotic disorder, may persist for 4 to 6 months. Indeed, some of these disorders continue in the long term even in the absence of further substance use, and a revised diagnosis (such as schizophrenia) may be made in those with long-persisting mental symptoms.

In terms of the features of individual substance-induced mental disorders, these are essentially the same as those of an independent mental disorder (a mood disorder or psychotic disorder, for example). There are no unique features of a substance-induced mental disorder. Likewise, all features which occur in the corresponding independent mental disorder can occur in a substance-induced mental disorder, though some are less common than others. For example, perceptual abnormalities or delusional thoughts with religiose content are somewhat unusual in a substance-induced psychotic disorder but are recognized.

Substance-Induced Neurocognitive Disorders

These disorders are primarily grouped within the Neurocognitive Disorders in ICD-11 but are cited in the chapter on substance use disorders, with a cross-reference provided.

Substance-Induced Amnestic Disorder is defined as memory impairment that is characterized by deficits in learning new information and/or the ability to recall previously learnt information. Recent memory is typically more disturbed than remote memory. The memory impairment is disproportionate to any impairment in other cognitive domains. When this is due to alcohol consumption, the eponymous diagnostic term 'Wernicke–Korsakoff syndrome' is applied.

Substance-Induced Dementia is defined as a global loss of cognitive function, characterized by persistent impairments in memory, language, and an ability to perform complex motor tasks. These features should meet the definitional requirements of dementia and be judged to be a direct consequence of substance use and to persist beyond the usual duration of intoxication or withdrawal.

An omission from ICD-11 is what many label as 'substance-related frontal lobe syndrome', or executive dysfunction. This comprises impairment in planning, decision-making, abstract thinking, and insight and is often accompanied by changes in personality and behaviours inappropriate to the circumstances. In ICD-10, this was accommodated, somewhat inappropriately, within 'Late-onset and Residual Psychotic Disorders'. In ICD-11 these syndromes are listed under the Dementia diagnosis, but with a requirement that the definitional requirements for dementia are fulfilled, which is typically not the case for this syndrome. More effort is required to define this syndrome, which is commonly seen in clinical practice, and to define its natural history.

Disorders Due to Use of Other Substances

The ICD-11 provides for the diagnosis of disorders due to other specified psychoactive substances (including medications) beyond the fourteen named substance (groups). Examples of these other substances include anabolic steroids, corticosteroids, antidepressants, anticholinergic medications, and antihistamines. All diagnoses that apply to the fourteen named substance (groups) are also applicable to these other psychoactive substances. For such substances not noted in ICD-11, the clinician may make a diagnosis where the clinical picture is compatible and where there is evidence a particular substance can produce a syndrome that is being diagnosed.

There is also provision in ICD-11 for the diagnosis of disorders due to non-psychoactive substances. These include laxatives, growth hormone, erythropoietin, certain proprietary and over-the-counter preparations, and folk remedies. Only two diagnoses may be made for substances in this latter category, namely, Harmful Pattern of Substance Use and Episode of Harmful Use. Substance Dependence is not allowed as a diagnosis. It would be expected that a diagnosis within one of the body organ/system chapters would also be made, for example peptic ulcer due to a non-steroidal anti-inflammatory drug or colonic motility disorder due to laxative use.

Subtypes and Qualifiers within ICD-11

For several diagnoses there are subtypes and qualifiers which offer a higher degree or precision in diagnosis according to the severity or course, or other manifestations of the disorder. For example, substance intoxication may be specified as (i) mild, (ii) moderate, or (iii) severe. Very severe intoxication, for example producing coma, is more typically included in the ICD-11 chapter on poisoning. A decision was made to exclude a fourth subtype of 'very severe' in favour of its location in the poisoning chapter. Substance Withdrawal may be specified as (i) with perceptual disturbances, (ii) with seizures, or (iii) with perceptual disturbances and seizures. There is no provision for specifying Substance Withdrawal as mild, moderate, or severe, given the constraints on the number of sub-categories imposed by the linear structure of ICD-11.

For the diagnosis of Substance Dependence, there are course qualifiers. These differ according to whether the substance is alcohol or something else, but in general encompass (i) ongoing (current) use of the substance, (ii) early full remission of 1 to 12 months' duration, (iii) sustained partial remission as evidenced by reduction in substance use for more than 12 months, and (iv) sustained full remission, defined as abstinence from the substance for more than 12 months.

Reactions to the ICD-11 Substance Diagnoses and Comments from Allen Frances

The response to the draft definitions and diagnostic guidelines issued in early 2019 and which underwent field testing though the network of WHO collaborating centres was overwhelmingly positive, with the major changes from ICD-10 being endorsed and with suggestions for adjusting some details in the guidelines being proposed – and largely accepted – leading to the final set of guidelines published in late 2021.

Because the definitive definitions and diagnostic guidelines were not published until late 2021, opportunity for empirical investigations at the time of writing has been limited. Chung and her colleagues[38] reported that in adolescents the prevalence of any alcohol or cannabis use disorder was lower according to the ICD-11 draft guidelines compared with DSM-5. Counterintuitively, ICD-11 alcohol and cannabis dependence were more common than the nearest equivalent diagnoses in DSM-5, namely, moderate/severe use disorder. An unresolved issue is how assessment questionnaires not developed for ICD-11 diagnoses perform as a method of capturing these diagnoses.

Following publication of the 2019 draft guidelines and a paper describing the development of these diagnoses (with particular reference to alcohol),[39] Rehm and his colleagues[40] critically reviewed whether the ICD-11 diagnoses had responded to several criticisms that had been levied against diagnostic and classification systems (both DSM and ICD). They posed several questions, which are listed below, together with responses from the present author:

- Did the new criteria include underlying brain processes?

  Brain processes, as emphasized in the RDoC criteria,[41] were comprehensively reviewed over the 15 years' developmental process of ICD-11 substance diagnoses. WHO issued a monograph in 2004. The underlying neurobiological processes are referred to in the definitions and diagnostic guidelines, being accepted as fundamental to the features of Substance Dependence, Substance Withdrawal, and the Substance-induced mental Disorders and Neurocognitive Disorders.

- Was the criticism regarding non-specific consequences remedied in the revision?

  As Rehm and colleagues note,[40] this criticism is mainly directed at the DSM-5 diagnostic criteria. ICD-11 does not accept non-specific consequences as grounds for making a substance disorders diagnosis. For Harmful Substance Use, there must be clear evidence (to the clinician) of physical and/or mental harm. Substance Dependence is not defined by harm but by evidence *inter alia* of increasing priority of substance use over time despite harm.

- Were the criteria changed to address issues of cultural specificity?

  ICD-11 eschews diagnoses which reflect social consequences as sufficient in themselves for the diagnosis of a substance use disorder. This long-standing stance has not been changed for ICD-11.

- Is the level of alcohol use adequately incorporated in the revision?

  The frequency and amount of alcohol (or other substance) use is the main basis for the diagnosis of Hazardous Substance Use. Harmful Use is defined by the occurrence of overt harm. Substance dependence is defined by evidence of a disorder of regulation of substance use and the three key features which are readily identified by clinicians.

- Have any attempts been made to close the gap between the two major classification system?

  It is true that DSM-5 diverged from DSM-IV, which almost overlapped with ICD-10 in the agreed features of Substance Dependence. WHO has a public health as well as a clinical orientation, and this is a key consideration for the diagnoses in the ICD system.

- Is it likely that the ICD-11 and its criteria will actually be used in clinical practice in primary care, where most patients with patterns of hazardous or harmful use or Alcohol Use Disorders (AUDs) first appear within the treatment system?

  Primary care versions of ICD-10 were prepared and are anticipated for ICD-11. The simplification of the diagnostic guidelines and inclusion of hazardous substance use have been taken to enhance its value for and facilitate uptake of the guidelines in primary care.

  ICD-11 has indeed added two new 'behavioural addictions', but these are Gambling Disorder and Gaming Disorder (i.e., a disorder due to playing online games). Compulsive sexual behaviour disorder is not conceptualized or listed as a behavioural addiction. Instead, it is in a separate section of ICD-11, as one of the impulse control disorders. It may be that the first few sentences of the ICD-11 description could be misinterpreted and so would be worth clarifying.

  In the ICD conceptualization of behavioural addictions, 'addiction' does not equate with 'passion'. There is a clear need for demonstrable impairment or harm to have occurred as a direct result of a pattern of gaming. Without evidence of harm, the diagnosis does not apply even if the other features (impaired control, increasing priority, and continued use despite harm) are fulfilled. I agree entirely with Frances' statement that 'behaviours shouldn't be counted as a mental disorder just because people derive a lot of pleasure and devote a lot of time to them'.

  With regard to his comments on Gaming Disorder, I agree with his comments about its increasingly negative impact. ICD-11 Gaming Disorder does not include people who like gaming but have it under control, not remotely.

  With regard to Gaming Disorder, the criteria of tolerance and withdrawal are not included as necessary criteria in ICD-11, and the reason is that there was, at the time the criteria were developed, insufficient scientific evidence that these were consistent occurrences in people who were considered to have Gaming Disorder. We were certainly aware of many media reports of suicidal feelings and acts of violence when gaming suddenly ceased, especially if this was enforced, but there was insufficient evidence for a coherent withdrawal syndrome (or of tolerance-like phenomena) at this time. However, tolerance and withdrawal are included in the description as 'additional clinical features', and so they are noted but not at an obligatory diagnostic level.

  The general point that precision in diagnostic criteria is vital and that we need to avoid diagnostic hyperinflation is well taken, but the way that the ICD diagnoses have been determined is fully in accord with this.

References

1. World Health Organization. (2018). *Global Status Report on Alcohol and Health 2018*. Geneva: World Health Organization. https://www.who.int/publications/i/item/9789241565639

2. World Health Organization. (2021). *WHO Report on the Global Tobacco Epidemic, 2021*. Geneva: World Health Organization.

3. GBD Risk Factors Collaborators. (2020). Global burden of 87 risk factors in 204 countries and territories, 1990–2019: a systematic analysis of the Global Burden of disease Study 2019. *Lancet*, **396**, 1223–1249.

4. United Nations Office on Drugs and Crime. (2021). *World Drug Report 2021*. Vienna: United Nations Office on Drugs and Crime.

5. Poznyak, V., Reed, G.M., Medina-Mora, M.E. (2018). Aligning the ICD-11 classification of disorders due to substance use with global service needs. *Epidemiol Psychiatr Sci*, **27**, 212–218.

6. World Health Organization. (2019). *International Classification of Diseases 11th Revision for Mortality and Morbidity Statistics (ICD-11 MMS)*. Geneva: World Health Organization. https://icd.who.int/browse11/l-m/en

7. World Health Organization. (2021). *International Classification of Diseases, 11th revision (ICD-11). Diagnostic Guidelines for Disorders Due to Substance Use*. Geneva: World Health Organization.

8. American Psychiatric Association. (2013). *Diagnostic and Statistical Manual of Mental Disorders (DSM-5)*, 5th ed. Washington, DC: American Psychiatric Association.

9. Saunders, J.B., Latt, N.C. (2020). Diagnostic definitions and classification of substance use disorders. In El-Guebaly, N. (Ed.), *Textbook of Addiction Treatment*, chapter 8. Springer.

10. World Health Organization. (2004). *Neuroscience of Psychoactive Substance Use and Dependence*. Geneva: World Health Organization.

11. Koob, G.F., Volkow, N.D. (2016). Neurobiology of addiction: a neurocircuitry analysis. *Lancet Psychiatry*, **3**, 760–773.

12. Saunders, J.B., Conigrave, K.M., Latt, N.C., et al. (2016). *Addiction Medicine*, 2nd ed. Oxford: Oxford University Press.

13. Room, R. (2006). Multicultural contexts and alcohol and drug use as symbolic behaviour. *Addict Res Theory*, **13**, 321–331.

14. World Health Organization. (1992). *ICD-10: International Statistical Classification of Diseases and Related Health Problems: Tenth Revision*. Geneva: World Health Organization.

15. World Health Organization. (1992). *The ICD-10 Classification of Mental and Behavioural Disorders: Clinical Descriptions and Diagnostic Guidelines*. Geneva: World Health Organization.

16. World Health Organization. (1993). *The ICD-10 Classification of Mental and Behavioural Disorders: Diagnostic Criteria for Research*. Geneva: World Health Organization.

17. Hasin, D., Grant, B.F., Cottler, L., et al. (1997). Nosological comparisons of alcohol and drug diagnoses: a multisite, multi-instrument international study. *Drug Alcohol Depend*, **47**, 217–226.

18. Pull, C.B., Saunders, J.B., Mavreas, V., et al. (1997). Concordance between ICD-10 alcohol and drug use disorder criteria and diagnoses as measured by the AUDADIS-ADR, CIDI and SCAN: results of a cross-national study. *Drug Alcohol Depend*, **47**, 207–216.

19. Poznyak, V. (2014). Background to the development of the section on Disorders due to Substance Use and Related Conditions in the draft ICD 11. Presented at the World Congress of the World Psychiatric Association, Madrid, Spain, September 2014. Available through the Department of Mental Health and Substance Abuse, World Health Organization, Geneva.

20. Saunders, J.B. (2014). Rationale for changes in the Clinical Descriptions and Diagnostic Guidelines of Disorders due to Substance Use and Related Conditions in the draft ICD 11. Presented at the World Congress of the World Psychiatric Association, Madrid, Spain, September 2014.

21. Reed, G.M., Rebello, T.J., Pike, K.M., et al. (2015). WHO's Global Clinical Practice Network for Mental Health. *Lancet Psychiatry*, **2**, 379–380.

22. Cottler, L.B., Grant, B.F. (2006). Characteristics of nosologically informative data sets that address key diagnostic issues facing the Diagnostic and Statistical Manual of Mental Disorders, fifth edition (DSM-V) and International Classification of Diseases, eleventh edition (ICD-11) substance use disorders workgroups. *Addiction*, **101**(Suppl 1), 161–169.

23. Saunders, J.B., Cottler L.B. (2007). The development of the Diagnostic and

Statistical Manual of Mental Disorders, Version V substance use disorders section: establishing the research framework. *Curr Opin Psychiatry*, **20**, 208–212.

24. Degenhardt, L., Bharat, C., Bruno, R., et al.; on behalf of the WHO World Mental Health Survey Collaborators. (2019). Concordance between the diagnostic guidelines for alcohol and cannabis use disorders in the draft ICD-11 and other classification systems: analysis of data from the WHO's World Mental Health Surveys. *Addiction*, **114**, 534–552.

25. Lago, L., Bruno, R., Degenhardt, L. (2016). Concordance of ICD-11 and DSM-5 definitions of alcohol and cannabis use disorders: a population survey. *Lancet Psychiatry*, **3**, 673–684.

26. Degenhardt, L., Bruno, R., Lintzeris, N., et al. (2015). Agreement between definitions of pharmaceutical opioid use disorders and dependence in people taking opioids for chronic non-cancer pain (POINT): a cohort study. *Lancet Psychiatry*, **2**, 314–322.

27. Edwards, G., Arif, A., Hodgson, R. (1981). Nomenclature and classification of drug and alcohol-related problems: a WHO memorandum. *Bull World Health Organ*, **59**, 255–242.

28. Paton A., Potter J.F., Saunders J.B. (1981). ABC of alcohol. Nature of the problem. *Br Med J*, **283**, 1318–1319.

29. Cherpitel, C.J., Ye, Y., Poznyak. V. (2018). Single episode of alcohol use resulting in injury: a cross-sectional study in 21 countries. *Bull World Health Organ*, **96**, 335–342.

30. Edwards, G., Gross, M.M. (1976). Alcohol dependence: provisional description of a clinical syndrome. *BMJ*, **1**, 1058–1061.

31. Gastfriend, D.R., Mee-Lee, D. (2004). The ASAM Patient Placement Criteria: context, concepts, and continuing development. *J Addict Dis*, **22**, 1–8.

32. MacMaster, S.A. (2004). Harm reduction: a new perspective on substance abuse services. *Soc Work*, **49**, 356–363.

33. Stocking, E., Hall, W.D., Lynskey, M., et al. (2016). Prevention, early intervention, harm reduction, and treatment of substance use in young people. *Lancet Psychiatry*, **3**, 280–296.

34. Wood, A.M., Kaptoge, S., Butterworth, A.S., et al. (2018). Risk thresholds for alcohol consumption: combined analysis of individual-participant data for 599 912 current drinkers in 83 prospective studies. *Lancet*, **391**, 1513–1523.

35. American Psychiatric Association. (1994). *Diagnostic and Statistical Manual of Mental Disorders*, 4th ed. (DSM-IV). Washington, DC: American Psychiatric Association.

36. American Psychiatric Association. (1987). *Diagnostic and Statistical Manual of Mental Disorders*, 3rd ed., Revised (DSM-III-R). Washington, DC: American Psychiatric Association.

37. Hasin, D.S., O'Brien, C.P., Auriacombe. M., et al. (2013). DSM-5 criteria for substance use disorders: recommendations and rationale. *Am J Psychiatry*, **170**, 834–851.

38. Chung, T., Cornelius, J., Clark. D., Martin, C. (2017). Greater prevalence of proposed ICD-11 alcohol and cannabis dependence compared to ICD-10, DSM-IV and DSM-5 in treated adolescents. *Alcohol Clin Exp Res*, **41**, 1584–1592.

39. Saunders, J.B., Degenhardt, L., Reed, G.M., Poznyak, V. (2019). Alcohol use disorders in ICD-11: past, present and future. *Alcohol Clin Exp Res*, **43**, 1617–1631.

40. Rehm, J., Heilig, M., Gual, A. (2019). ICD-11 for alcohol use disorders: not a convincing answer to the challenges. *Alcohol Clin Exp Res*, **43**, 2296–2300.

41. Insel, T., Cuthbert, B., Garvey, M., et al. (2010). Research Domain Criteria (RDoC): toward a new classification framework for research on mental disorders. *Am J Psychiatry*, **167**, 748–751.

Chapter 7

Child and Adolescent Psychiatric Disorders

M. Elena Garralda

Introduction

The most important change in ICD-11 for child and adolescent psychiatry has been the loss of the group devoted to specific disorders of childhood. Instead, and in recognition of the lifespan nature of many psychiatric disorders, those that present in children and young people are included with all other disorders, and these apply across *all ages*. To assist interpretation, there are additional clauses relevant to childhood presentations in ICD-11.

Two groups of disorders with an onset that is typically shown in childhood are described in the chapter Neurodevelopmental and Dissocial/Disruptive Disorders. Both are aligned with their corresponding DSM-5 categories, but there are some differences. The main innovations in neurodevelopmental disorders are the inclusion and renaming of Mental Retardation (now termed Disorders of Intellectual Development) and Hyperkinetic Disorder (now Attention Deficit Hyperactivity Disorder or ADHD).

There are also refinements that have followed changes in practice and research. Pervasive Developmental Disorders in ICD-10 are now renamed Autistic Spectrum Disorders or ASD. There have also been modifications to the Disruptive Behaviour & Dissocial Disorder group – which now includes Oppositional Defiant Disorder (ODD) and Conduct Dissocial Disorders (CDD).

As Geoffrey Reed pointed out in the first chapter of this book, many categories of disorder have been replaced by a set of symptom *qualifier* ratings that much better describe the patient's functioning on several dimensions. Irritability has been introduced for Oppositional Defiant Disorder, age of onset (childhood vs adolescence) for Conduct Disorder, and low prosocial behaviour for both.

Neurodevelopmental & Disruptive Behaviour and Dissocial Disorders

For all disorders in this section, those included are expected to create sufficient adversity to result in 'significant impairment in personal, family, social, educational, or other important areas of functioning'.

Neurodevelopmental Disorders

Neurodevelopmental Disorders in ICD-11 include the noticeable presence of behavioural and cognitive problems during the developmental period (i.e., prior to 18 years of age). These encompass difficulties with intellectual, motor, language, and social functions. They can be differentiated from other disorders that also display neurodevelopmental features such as schizophrenia, because in developmental disorders these features are central to the disorder. Although it has long been presumed that brain changes underlie neurodevelopmental disorders, the aetiology is likely to be complex and largely remains unknown. In our present state of knowledge, developmental disorders cannot be explained by diseases of the nervous system, by sensory or purely environmental (social, cultural/ethnic) hazards, or by intellectual deficits or other neurodevelopment disorders, even allowing for the considerable co-morbidity that exists between them.

The main categories in this group are Disorders of Intellectual Development; Specific Developmental Disorders (primarily affecting speech/language, learning, or motor/movement); and Autism Spectrum and Attention Deficit Hyperactivity Disorders.

The essential features of the main categories (except for the Disorders of Intellectual Development, which are covered in Chapter 10 by Cooper and Kogan) are described here in the following sections.

Specific Developmental Disorders

Speech or Language Disorders: difficulties in understanding and/or producing verbal speech or language, and problems in using language to communicate with others. They are separated into different categories, but there is a considerable degree of overlap between the different speech and language disorders.

a) Developmental Speech Sound Disorders (errors of pronunciation, articulation, or phonology). These may be associated with dysfunction of the mouth and swallowing and with early feeding difficulties.

b) Developmental Speech Fluency Disorder (disruption of the normal rhythmic flow and rate of speech). This includes stuttering and stammering, often begins in childhood and adolescence, and is commonly associated with social anxiety.

c) Developmental Language Disorder with persistent deficits in the acquisition, understanding, production, or use of language, spoken or signed. This may include phonological awareness (the ability to recognize and manipulate the spoken parts of sentences and words), syntax, morphology, grammar, semantics, narrative discourse, and pragmatics. It can manifest as marked discrepancy between verbal and non-verbal ability, often runs in families, and is sometimes a presenting feature in individuals with specific chromosomal anomalies.

Its three *qualifiers* are impairments of 1) receptive and expressive language; 2) expressive language; 3) pragmatic language (i.e., difficulties understanding and using language in social contexts, such as making inferences and understanding verbal humour).

When there is an underlying neurological cause, speech and language disorders are to be diagnosed as Secondary Speech or Language Syndrome.

Developmental Learning Disorder: this describes limitations in learning academic skills of reading, writing, or arithmetic. It covers a group of conditions that may involve impaired psychological processes such as phonological processing, memory, executive functions, and perceptual/motor integration. It has specific *qualifiers* for primary problems with reading, mathematics, or written expression.

Developmental Motor Co-ordination Disorder: with significant delay in the acquisition of gross or fine motor skills and impairment in the execution of coordinated motor skills (i.e., clumsiness, slowness, or inaccuracy of motor performance). It involves a delay in achieving the motor milestones of crawling, standing, walking, and running (gross functioning), or writing, manipulation, and other fine hand or finger movements (fine motor function).

Stereotyped Movement Disorder: voluntary, repetitive, stereotyped movements, not caused by substance or medication ingestion; *qualifiers*: with and without self-injury.

Primary Tics or Tic Disorders: include several categories, Tourette Syndrome, Chronic Motor Tic Disorder, and Chronic Phonic Tic Disorder. They are classified with Diseases of the Nervous System (ICD-11, Chapter 8), but cross-listed with the Neurodevelopmental Disorders because of high co-occurrence and familial association. All share an onset during the developmental period, and symptoms must be present for at least 1 year. They include (1) Tourette syndrome: combination of motor and phonic tics, not secondary to a medical condition, (2) Chronic motor tic disorder: persistent motor tics, and (3) Chronic phonic tic disorder: persistent phonic tics.

Boundaries with Normality and Other Disorders

Children vary considerably in the sequence and age at which they acquire developmental skills such as speech and language, or display symptoms such as tics; repetitive stereotyped movements such as thumb sucking are not uncommonly transiently present in childhood. In developmental disorders, the delays or symptoms are marked and persistent and cause problems and significant limitations in children's abilities.

Differential diagnosis will include intellectual disability and other neurodevelopmental disorders, selective mutism or obsessive–compulsive disorders, sensory impairments, and neurodegenerative or other disorders of the nervous system or other medical conditions.

Autistic Spectrum Disorders

The two essential criteria for the diagnosis of this condition are:

a) Persistent deficits in initiating and sustaining social communication and reciprocal social interactions that are outside the expected range of typical functioning, after taking into account the individual's age and level of intellectual development.
b) Persistent restricted, repetitive, inflexible patterns of behaviour; interests or activities that are clearly atypical or excessive for the individual's age, gender, and sociocultural context; lifelong, excessive, and persistent hypersensitivity or hyposensitivity to sensory stimuli.

The three *qualifiers* to Autistic Spectrum Disorders are (1) co-occurrence with disorders of intellectual development, (2) the degree of functional language impairment (none or mild; impaired; complete absence), and (3) the presence or absence of loss of previously acquired skills.

The term 'spectrum' in Autism Spectrum Disorders refers to the wide range of symptoms and severity, the presentation varying with age and intellectual ability. It is common in young children for parents and schools to first become aware of intellectual or other developmental delays. At a later stage in childhood, behaviour or social problems may cause concern and arouse the attention of services, especially school. In adolescence, anxiety and depression may often be presenting features. Some individuals, not at the extreme end of the spectrum, can function adequately, and sometimes excel, by making an exceptional effort to compensate for symptoms or being able to manoeuvre their environments to places where social interaction is kept to a minimum. Often, cognitive skills are patchy, and some individuals show marked ability in some areas but very impaired ability in others. Autistic Spectrum Disorder is sometimes associated with epilepsy and catatonic states. Genetic disorders, particularly Fragile X syndrome (FXS), Cornelia de Lange syndrome (CdLS), and tuberous sclerosis, have been noted to have links to autism.

Boundaries with Normality and Other Disorders
Typically, developing individuals vary in their social interaction and communication skills and in their engagement in repetitive and stereotyped behaviours. But in autism there is a marked and persistent deviation from skills and behaviours expected in relation to the person's age, gender, intellectual functioning, and sociocultural context. ICD-11's ASD has incorporated into its spectrum the earlier ICD-10 diagnosis (F84) of Asperger syndrome, indicative of autism in individuals without intellectual disability.

Differential diagnosis includes not only other neurodevelopmental disorders, but also a range of disorders such as oppositional/defiant, food, anxiety and obsessive–compulsive, schizophrenia, and attachment- and personality-related disorders, as well as medical conditions including diseases of the nervous system.

Attention Deficit Hyperactivity Disorder (ADHD)

ADHD describes a persistent pattern (with a duration of at least 6 months) of inattention and/or a combination of hyperactivity and impulsivity symptoms outside the limits of normal variation as expected for age and level of intellectual development. Symptoms vary according to chronological age and disorder severity. The three qualifiers are: (1) those of predominant inattention, (2) those of hyperactive-impulsive behaviour, and (3) the combined presence of both. The manifestations and severity of ADHD often vary according to the demands of different environments, particularly school and home. It often places a limit on academic achievement. For the diagnosis to be made in adult life, symptoms should have been present before age 12, and corroborating evidence from school records or informants is expected. The acute onset of hyperactive behaviour in a school-age child or adolescent should raise the possibility of another mental disorder or medical condition.

Boundaries with Normality and Other Disorders
Diagnosis should only be made when there is clear evidence of the severity, pervasiveness, and persistence of symptoms, and consequent impairment.

Differential diagnosis includes other neuro-developmental and/or potential co-morbid disorders, including anxiety/fear-related and personality disorders, conduct/dissocial/substance use disorders, the effects of certain prescribed medications (often a hidden association), and attentional symptoms due to other medical conditions.

Disruptive Behaviour and Dissocial Disorders

The essential feature of these disorders is the expression of persistent behaviour problems across multiple settings, with onset occurring most commonly in childhood. The behaviours range from disruptive challenging behaviour such as marked defiance, disobedience, and spitefulness, to more serious antisocial violations of the basic rights of others or of societal norms or laws. They are frequently associated with deprived psychosocial environments such as family or peer group dysfunction, and with poor school or work performance.

Oppositional Defiant Disorder

This condition describes a persistent pattern lasting at least 6 months in which unusually marked defiant, disobedient, and provocative behaviour is shown. This often co-occurs with persistently angry or irritable mood. It is usually first shown in early childhood when there is headstrong, argumentative, and provocative behaviour without much in the way of stimulus. It creates significant impairment in several areas of functioning and, importantly, is diffuse in its presentation, and not accounted for by a specific relationship between the individual and a particular authority figure.

The features of irritability and anger may reflect a degree of mood dysregulation and sometimes predominate, but these alone are not sufficient to make a diagnosis. Some individuals may present with limited prosocial emotions. There is often conflict in relationships with family members and this can lead to poor social supports. It can co-occur with neurodevelopmental and other psychiatric disorders.

The *qualifiers* of oppositional defiant disorder are (1) with and without chronic irritability and anger and (2) with or without limited prosocial emotions (callous, unemotional traits, such as limited empathy or sensitivity, remorse, shame, or guilt).

Boundaries with Normality and Other Disorders

Oppositional Defiant Disorder should be differentiated from defiant, disobedient, and irritable behaviours within the boundaries of expected behaviour.

Differential diagnosis includes Conduct/Dissocial and Personality Disorders, Attention Deficit Hyperactivity and Autistic Spectrum Disorders, Mood, Anxiety or Fear-Related Disorders, and Intermittent Explosive Disorder.

Conduct–Dissocial Disorder

Conduct–dissocial disorder (CDD) is characterized by a repetitive and persistent pattern of fundamentally antisocial behaviour whereby the basic rights of others are violated, the disruption created is outside the range of social or cultural norms, and the rules and laws of society are broken. The behaviour includes aggression towards others, bullying, cruelty, stealing, destruction of property, deceitfulness, and theft, and, in adolescents, repeated staying out late, running away, drug misuse, and skipping school (truancy). It can co-occur with neurodevelopmental and a number of other psychiatric disorders.

Qualifiers include (1) childhood onset (features present before 10 years of age) versus adolescent onset (features do not present before 10 years); and (2) with or without limited prosocial emotions. In adolescence in particular, the behaviour may be manifest within a delinquent peer group. It frequently co-occurs with oppositional defiant disorder and not uncommonly with a number of neurodevelopmental and other psychiatric disorders. Individuals with limited prosocial emotions and those with childhood onset are at greater risk for more persistent and severe antisocial behaviour and of developing personality disorder later in life. But it is important to note that the age of onset subtype and the prosocial emotions qualifier are distinct and should be considered separately.

Boundaries with Normality and Other Disorders
Conduct–Dissocial Disorder should be differentiated from activities such as engaging in political protest and criminal offences.

Differential Diagnosis: It should also be differentiated from Oppositional Defiant, Attention Deficit Hyperactivity, and Mood Disorders; from Intermittent Explosive, Personality; and disorders due to substance use.

Changes from Close or Equivalent ICD-10 Disorders

A key change in ICD-11 in relation to ICD-10 is the elimination of Behavioural and Emotional Disorders with onset usually occurring in childhood and adolescence (F90–F98), affected by the emotional and behavioural immaturities of childhood: these have been distributed across all-age disorders with which they share symptoms, and which now mention any specific variations in child presentations.

There have also been a number of changes in terminology of both disorder groups and individual disorders.

The *multi-axial framework* of prior versions of ICD and DSM has been discarded. This was popular in child psychiatric practice, as it allowed the classification of common co-morbidities between psychiatric and neurodevelopmental and medical disorders, as well as with psychosocial contributory factors. However, ICD-11 allows instead the diagnosis of all types of co-morbidities, which also obviates the diagnosis of interface disorders such as ICD-10 'Mixed disorders of conduct and emotions'.

The Redistribution of Specific ICD-10 Childhood Categories

The loss of the Emotional Disorders with onset specific to Childhood (F93) means that childhood disorders such as Separation Anxiety Disorder and Selective Mutism are now diagnosed with the all-age 'Anxiety and Fear-Related disorders'.

The Feeding disorders of childhood have become part of a new 'Feeding and Eating Disorders' group, which incorporates the new and childhood-relevant 'Avoidant/restrictive food intake disorder' or ARFID. Enuresis and Encopresis make up the new ICD-11 'Elimination Disorders' group.

ICD-10's Disorders of social functioning with onset specific to childhood and adolescence (F94) included Reactive attachment and Disinhibited attachment disorders of childhood. These have now found a home with the 'Disorders specifically associated with stress' as 'Reactive attachment disorder' and 'Disinhibited social engagement disorder'.

ICD-10's Conduct Disorders (F91) have become ICD-11's 'Disruptive and Dissocial Disorders' and the Mixed disorders of conduct and emotions (F92) have been discontinued.

Neurodevelopmental Disorders

By and large, ICD-10's Disorders of Psychological Development are included under ICD-11 'Neurodevelopmental Disorders'. An important change is the substitution of ICD-10 Pervasive Developmental Disorders by 'Autistic Spectrum disorders': this includes the earlier Pervasive Developmental, Asperger Syndrome, and Atypical Autism categories. Rett Syndrome and Disintegrative Disorder have been moved to the Diseases of the Nervous System causing Regression. The main changes in the neurodevelopmental disorders group are noted in Table 7.1.

Table 7.1 ICD-10 Disorders of Psychological Development & ICD-11 Neurodevelopmental Disorders

ICD-10	ICD-11
Disorders of psychological development	**Neurodevelopmental Disorders**
a. Specific developmental disorders	
-of speech & language/communication	-of speech and language
-of scholastic skills/learning	-of learning
-of motor function	-developmental motor coordination
	-stereotyped movement disorder
	-tic disorders (Disorders of Nervous System) (cross-listed here)
b. Disorders of social development, communication and behaviour	
Pervasive developmental disorders	Autistic spectrum disorders
c. Other disorders	
Mental retardation	Disorders of Intellectual Development
Hyperkinetic disorders	Attention Deficit Hyperactivity Disorder
-----	Secondary Neurodevelopmental syndrome
Neurodevelopmental syndrome	

Comparison with DSM-5 Equivalent Diagnoses

The disorders addressed in this chapter are generally aligned in DSM-5 and ICD-11, but there are some differences worthy of note. Both systems have introduced diagnostic sub-categories (*specifiers* in DSM-5 and *qualifiers* in ICD-11) but these are not always coterminous or in line with each other. Differences between the two diagnostic systems are discussed here.

Neurodevelopmental Disorders

Developmental Language Disorder

Both ICD-11 Developmental Language Disorder and DSM-5 Language Disorder involve deficits in the acquisition and use of intrinsic language skills such as sentence structure and vocabulary, but ICD-11 also includes a pragmatic deficit or 'the ability to understand and use language in social contexts, for example making inferences, understanding verbal humour and resolving ambiguous meaning'.

A pragmatic language deficit in ICD-11 will trigger the Developmental Language Disorder *pragmatic language qualifier*. In contrast, individuals with pragmatic language deficits *who do not display other autistic features* are diagnosed in DSM-5 as having a distinct Social (Pragmatic) Communication Disorder. The ICD-11 working group considered there was insufficient evidence for this new disorder, given that most children with pragmatic language deficits can be diagnosed as having another language or an autistic disorder.

Autism Spectrum Disorder

The diagnostic criteria in ICD-11 and DSM-5 are similar and both regard autism as a spectrum. However, DSM-5 is more descriptive of the deficits required, and the examples of 'restricted, repetitive and inflexible patterns' of behaviour in ICD-11 are more characteristic of individuals with autism *without* intellectual disability than those in DSM-5.

Attention Deficit Hyperactivity Disorder (ADHD)

The ICD-11 and DSM-5 diagnostic requirements are broadly comparable, but DSM-5 is more prescriptive in specifying a precise symptom count requirement for diagnosis. In addition, ICD-11 has added 'impulsive responding without consideration of risks or consequences' as a likely adult manifestation of the disorder. And whilst for adult diagnosis both systems require that manifestations of ADHD be present by age 12 years, ICD-11 also asks for evidence of significant inattention and/or hyperactivity–impulsivity symptoms prior to that age, DSM-5 simply requiring that 'several symptoms' have been present in childhood.

Disruptive/Dissocial Disorders

Both classifications include Oppositional Defiant and Conduct Disorders under Disruptive/Dissocial Disorders, but the DSM-5 categorization is broader in that it also includes Impulse Control Disorders under the rubric of Disruptive, Impulse Control and Conduct Disorders, and there are differences in disorder terminology. ICD-11 Impulse Control Disorders include Compulsive Sexual Behaviour Disorders and Secondary Impulse Control Syndrome, whilst DSM-5 includes Other Specific Disruptive Disorders or Personality Change due to another medical condition.

Another difference concerns *qualifiers*: the new sub-category *with limited prosocial emotions* is applied to both ODD and Conduct Disorder in ICD-11, but applies only to Conduct Disorder in DSM-5.

Oppositional Defiant Disorder

An important distinction between the two systems is the introduction of an *irritability qualifier* in ICD-11. In addition to argumentative/defiant behaviour and vindictiveness, angry/irritable moods and behaviours (tempers, being easily annoyed, often angry and resentful) are symptoms of ODD in both classification systems. However, only ICD-11 has introduced a *chronic irritability/anger qualifier*. This is based on the research evidence for such a separate construct, and on the specific associations of the irritability dimension of ODD in clinic-referred boys with a continuous pattern of mood and anxiety symptoms through adolescence and young adulthood.

To conceptualize this group of clinically impaired angry/irritable children, DSM-5 has created a new disorder called Disruptive mood dysregulation disorder or DMDD, listed in the Depressive Disorders chapter. The ICD-11 working group considered that there was insufficient evidence for a separate DMDD because of limited reliability, lack of psychiatric consensus, and high rates of overlap with other disorders, particularly Oppositional Defiant Disorder.

Advantages of ICD-11 Classification

The classification of child psychiatric disorders remains crucial to communication between all those involved with services, a tool for communication by clinicians, families, researchers, and policy makers. Classification is increasingly a requirement for service function and development across different countries.

Whilst earlier hopes for a clinico-pathological aetiological approach to diagnosis have not been realized, the changes made in ICD-11 including the detailed disorder descriptions – based as much as possible on existing practice and research findings – and the harmonization with DSM-5 will contribute to enhancing communication between different stakeholders.

Central to the development of ICD-11 and DSM-5 was an overall philosophy of reducing the number of psychiatric disorders, leaving the best validated and found to be clinically helpful. An example in the neurodevelopmental disorders group is the amalgamation of several ICD-10 Pervasive Developmental Disorders into one Autistic Spectrum Disorder group with separate qualifiers.

The lifespan approach has meant the redistribution of previously child-specific disorders of childhood. Grouping feeding disorders of childhood with adult eating disorders has been justified by existing evidence of links between feeding problems in infancy and anorexia and bulimia nervosa. Overall, the lifespan strategy acknowledges the fact that a considerable percentage of adult psychiatric disorders are already manifest in childhood and adolescence. Applying the same diagnostic criteria across the age range for problems such as depressive disorders helps guide and focus the assessment and management of affected children and young people who in earlier ICD versions may have been diagnosed as having non-specific emotional disorders of childhood. One further advantage of the lifespan approach is that it may facilitate the recognition and management of underlying neurodevelopmental disorders in adults presenting with a variety of psychiatric disorders.

Impairment of function is now a key feature for diagnoses. This has been challenged on the grounds that non-symptomatic but treatable medical anomalies such as hypertension constitute treatable medical problems. Hypertension, however, may be regarded as a risk factor rather than a disorder itself. Lack of impairment does not entail lack of mental health difficulty, nor does it preclude the introduction of appropriate preventive interventions, but it does help set a useful threshold for clarifying and seeking the level of specialist intervention required.

The introduction of co-morbidity and of disorder *qualifiers* is important for child and adolescent psychiatric practice, especially following the removal of previous multi-axial classifications. It allows the recognition of complexity and is highly relevant to management planning.

The ICD-11 *qualifiers* provide useful additional information of relevance to prognosis and management. This is clearly the case for intellectual disability and language problems qualifiers in autism and for low prosocial emotions in children with conduct disorders. Links between childhood irritability and later mood disorders in some children with Oppositional Defiant Disorder are similarly acknowledged by a *qualifier*. This may serve as a reminder of the need for careful differential diagnosis from anxiety or other psychiatric disorders in children presenting with irritability, a ubiquitous symptom amongst clinic referrals. In addition, some *qualifiers* allow for the identification of disorder severity levels, which is again of relevance for treatment and service involvement.

In clinical practice, the detailed ICD-11 CDDGs (Clinical Descriptions and Diagnostic Guidelines) can act as both a helpful memory aid and a mini-textbook. CDDGs have been guided by the principle of clinical utility, to aid clinical encounters, and to be globally applicable and scientifically valid.

Discussion

The recognition of co-morbidity in ICD-11 helps to document the complexity of a number of problems seen by Child and Adolescent Mental Health Services (CAMHS). It also points towards the need to promote research into common risk factors, which in turn may lead to redefinition of disorders. This is particularly relevant for the neurodevelopmental disorders.

Future work might help clarify and disentangle the nature of other co-morbidities throughout ICD-11. For example, it is likely that personality disorder in some individuals will be an adult manifestation and consequence of neurodevelopmental problems. A child with an autistic disorder might present in adulthood with personality disorder with predominant anankastic and detachment features. Children with early dissocial and disruptive disorders may present in adulthood with features of a personality disorder with dissocial features. Future research may help clarify the extent of their developmental congruence and shared underlying risks.

There is currently debate on whether certain disorders of childhood such as ICD-11's Reactive attachment and Disinhibited Social Engagement Disorders should be best conceptualized as the result of developmental trauma – which would be in line with the fact that ICD-11 groups them under 'Disorders Specifically Associated with Stress' – or whether they should be understood within a neurodevelopmental perspective. This again is likely to generate research to clarify relationships.

It would be wrong to assume that the ICD-11 classification will be embraced with enthusiasm overall. The intention of a good classification is to promote improved communication, to inform management and document service data, and to lead to better care. But it is acknowledged that the use of psychiatric categories to define children's problems is not universally popular with CAMHS practitioners. CAMHS usually involve multidisciplinary teams with clinicians holding complementary but also alternative perspectives on children's problems. Some clinicians are both uncomfortable and unskilled in the use of classification, or actively oppose it, choosing not to 'label' children with any diagnosis. These practitioners, many of whom are enthusiastic and caring, are concerned about the potential of diagnosis as a source of stigma. They advocate an approach that focuses on understanding and modifying troubled children's inner worlds or difficulties in the family or broader environment, regardless of diagnosis, and may use sociocultural arguments to support their policies.

They are right to conclude that environmental factors are highly relevant in the genesis of child psychiatric disorders, and it is fair to add that many CAMHS interventions are non-specific and trans-diagnostic. Nevertheless, unless there is greater familiarity with ICD-11 in CAMHS multidisciplinary teams, there is potential for confusion and slower development towards a common approach to nomenclature and both the provision of helpful feedback to families and service data.

Diagnosis in child psychiatry is normally supplemented by a formulation of the problem, indicating how a particular disorder developed and how it affects an individual child, taking into account biological, developmental, and environmental risk and protective factors. These are further conceptualized as predisposing, precipitant, and maintaining factors of the disorder. But a formulation is not normally a substitute for a diagnosis, and the ICD-11 introduction of the severity of other qualifiers for some disorders can be helpful in backing up formulations.

The psychiatric disorders described in ICD-11 represent the first attempt to join up the classification of child, adolescent, and adult conditions into a single system. This, as a first attempt, is bound to be imperfect, and thus will need to adapt and change in the light of new knowledge and expertise. The goal remains one of integrating knowledge, promoting better communication between all those involved in care, and opening the way for a new and better understanding and management of mental health problems. ICD-11 is still not far off the starting block in this respect, but the knowledge and expertise supporting its psychiatric categories can be regarded as a welcome step forward.

Background Reading

Evans, S.C., Burke, J.D., Roberts, M.C., et al. (2017). Irritability in child and adolescent psychopathology: an integrative review for ICD-11. *Clin Psychol Rev*, **53**, 29–45.

Evans, S.C., Roberts, M.C., Keeley, J.W., et al. (2020). Diagnostic classification of irritability and oppositionality in youth: a global field study comparing ICD-11 with ICD-10 and DSM-5. *J Child Psychol Psychiatry*, **62**, 303–312.

First, M.B., Gaebel, W., Maj, M., et al. (2021). An organization- and category-level comparison of diagnostic requirements for mental disorders in ICD-11 and DSM-5. *World Psychiatry*, **20**, 34–51.

Fristad, M.A. (2020). Commentary: what to do with irritability? Do not give it a new diagnostic home—a commentary on Evans et al (2020). *J Child Psychol Psychiatry*, **62**, 313–315.

Garralda, M.E. (2016). ICD-11 – comparison with DSM-5 and implications for child & adolescent psychiatric disorders. In Hodes, M. & Gau, S. (Eds.), *Positive Mental Health, Fighting Stigma and Promoting Resiliency for Children and Adolescents*, pp. 15–35. London: Academic Press/Elsevier.

Lochman, J.E., Evans, S.C., Burke, J.D., et al. (2015). An empirically based alternative to DSM-5's disruptive mood dysregulation disorder for ICD-11. *World Psychiatry*, **14**, 30–33.

Reed, G.M., First, M.B., Kogan, C.S., et al. (2019). Innovations and changes in the ICD-11 classification of mental, behavioural and neurodevelopmental disorders. *World Psychiatry*, **18**, 3–19.

Reed, G.M., Keeley, J.W., Rebello, T.J., et al. (2018). Clinical utility of ICD-11 diagnostic guidelines for high-burden mental disorders: results from mental health settings in 13 countries. *World Psychiatry*, **17**, 306–315.

Robles, R., de la Pena, F., Medina-Mora, M.E., et al. (2021). ICD-11 guidelines for mental and behavioral disorders of children and adolescents: reliability and clinical utility. *Psychiatr Serv*, **73**(4), 396–402. https://doi.org/10.1176/appi.ps.202000830

Rutter, M. (2011). Research Review: child psychiatric diagnosis and classification: concepts, findings, challenges and potential. *J Child Psychol Psychiatry*, **52**, 647–660.

Tyrer, P., Reed, G.M., Crawford, M.J. (2015). Classification, assessment, prevalence, and effect of personality disorder. *Lancet*, **385**, 717–726.

Uher, R., Rutter, M. (2012). Classification of feeding and eating disorders: review of evidence and proposals for ICD-11. *World Psychiatry*, **11**, 80–92.

Chapter 8

Anxiety and Fear-Related Disorders and Obsessive–Compulsive and Related Disorders

Dan J. Stein, Cary S. Kogan, & Christine Lochner

Anxiety and Fear-Related Disorders and Obsessive-Compulsive and Related Disorders are two new groupings in the Mental, Behavioural or Neurodevelopmental Disorders chapter of ICD-11. Anxiety and Fear-Related Disorders comprises generalized anxiety disorder, panic disorder, agoraphobia, specific phobia, social anxiety disorder, separation anxiety disorder, and selective mutism. Substance-induced anxiety disorders, hypochondriasis, and secondary anxiety syndrome are also cross-listed. Obsessive-Compulsive and Related Disorders comprises obsessive-compulsive disorder, body dysmorphic disorder, olfactory reference disorder, hypochondriasis (health anxiety disorder), hoarding disorder, and body-focused repetitive behaviour disorders. Substance-induced and secondary obsessive-compulsive and related disorders, and Tourette syndrome, are also cross-listed.

This chapter reviews key aspects of the two new groupings and their component disorders. We begin with a brief discussion of the ICD-11 meta-structure, before moving on to a consideration of each of these groupings.

Meta-Structure of Anxiety and Obsessive-Compulsive Disorders

A series of workshops were held in preparation for developing DSM-5, included specific meetings on fear-circuitry disorders[1] and obsessive-compulsive and related disorders.[2] At that early point, there was a great deal of interest in developing a neuroscientifically grounded nosology that included a focus on laboratory-based behavioural dimensions.[3-5] Research on anxiety disorders has emphasized the potential role of fear conditioning in the aetiology of these conditions, has investigated fear circuitry including amygdala-related pathways in animal and human anxiety, and has suggested that fear extinction may play a role in the treatment of fear-circuitry disorders.[1] This kind of work suggests the diagnostic validity of a grouping of anxiety and fear-related disorders in the classification system.[6]

Research on obsessive-compulsive disorder (OCD), on the other hand, has suggested that this condition is characterized by deficits in cognitive control, with a shift from goal-directed to habit-driven behaviour that is underpinned by alterations in frontal cortico-striatal-thalamic-cortical (CSTC) circuitry.[7,8] Such work has provided a basis for differentiating OCD from other anxiety disorders, for linking OCD with other conditions characterized by alterations in habit-driven behaviour (e.g., body-focused repetitive behavioural disorders such as trichotillomania), and for suggesting that specific interventions that normalize CSTC circuitry (e.g., exposure therapy and response prevention and high-dose serotonin reuptake inhibitors (SRIs)) may be useful in different Obsessive-Compulsive and Related Disorders

(OCRDs). This kind of research suggests the diagnostic validity of this grouping in the classification system.[7,8]

An early review by the DSM-5 Anxiety, Obsessive-Compulsive Spectrum, Posttraumatic, and Dissociative Disorders Workgroup found that there was considerable overlap of validators across OCD and the anxiety disorders, and recommended a grouping termed 'Anxiety and Obsessive-Compulsive Disorders'.[9] This proposal was seen as recognizing that anxiety disorders and OCRDs had important overlaps and differences. There were, however, several moving parts to these discussions, with debate around whether generalized anxiety disorder (GAD) and post-traumatic stress disorder (PTSD) belonged in the anxiety disorders.[10] The final DSM-5 decision was to retain GAD in anxiety disorders, to have new categories on OCRDs and Trauma and Stressor-Related Disorders, and to list these categories adjacent to one another, given their relatedness.[11]

The ICD-11 developers were particularly focused on improving clinical utility of the classification.[12] From an ICD-11 perspective, introducing groupings of Anxiety and Fear-Related Disorders, and Obsessive-Compulsive and Related Disorders (OCRDs) was useful in reminding clinicians of the importance of considering these conditions (as they are often underdiagnosed and undertreated), to ask patients with any one of these conditions about the presence of another (OCRDs, for example, are more often co-morbid with one another than with other conditions), and to consider the use of similar evaluation measures in each grouping (such as the Yale–Brown Obsessive-Compulsive Rating Scale for a number of different OCRDS) as well as similar intervention methods (such as fear extinction for anxiety disorders, and exposure and response prevention for OCRDs).[6,8]

Diagnostic validity underpins clinical utility, and certainly DSM-5 considered issues of clinical utility, while ICD-11 considered issues of diagnostic validity. Still, the different weighting given to these considerations, and ICD-11's concern with global applicability, contributed in part to some of their differences.[13] In addition, ICD-11 allows for cross-listing of conditions, and several conditions in the ICD-11 grouping of OCRDs are also listed elsewhere. Thus, ICD-11 takes a broader approach to the OCRDs than does DSM-5 by also including olfactory reference disorder (which is particularly common in the East),[14] hypochondriasis (cross-listed in Anxiety and Fear-Related Disorders), and Tourette syndrome (cross-listed in Neurodevelopmental Disorders and in Movement Disorders).

Anxiety and Fear-Related Disorders

Anxiety and Fear-Related Disorders in ICD-11 are all characterized by excessive anxiety or fear, but each has a different focus of apprehension.[6] Most of these conditions were classified by ICD-10 in the Neurotic, Stress-Related, and Somatoform Disorders grouping. The focus of apprehension may be highly specific (e.g., in specific phobia), may relate to a wider range of situations (e.g., in social anxiety disorder), or may be characterized by general apprehensiveness (e.g., in generalized anxiety disorder). The Anxiety and Fear-Related Disorders are also characterized by varying degrees of physiological arousal and of behavioural avoidance. The ICD-11 takes a lifespan approach to psychopathology; thus, the grouping does not separate childhood from adult disorders but rather provides information on the developmentally distinct presentations of included disorders.

A first step of the ICD-11 Working Group on the Classification of Mood and Anxiety Disorders was to review the literature on the Anxiety and Fear-Related Disorders, with a particular focus on clinical utility and global applicability.[6] Next, the WHO's Global Practice Network was employed to assess the diagnostic accuracy and clinical utility of proposed ICD-11 diagnostic guidelines. Diagnostic accuracy and clinical utility of ICD-11 diagnostic guidelines for Anxiety and Fear-Related Disorders were equivalent or superior to those of ICD-10.[17] However, clinicians had difficulty with distinguishing the boundary between disorder and normality for sub-threshold cases of anxiety, which is perhaps consistent with how difficult this boundary can be in daily practice. Use of the ICD-11 guidelines for Obsessive-Compulsive and Related Disorders also resulted in more accurate diagnosis of case vignettes compared with the ICD-10 guidelines, particularly in differentiating OCRD presentations from one another.[18]

In addition, a field study comprising 28 participating centres in 13 countries found that inter-rater reliability on the ICD-11 diagnostic guidelines for Anxiety and Fear-Related disorders was moderate to high, with kappa coefficients ranging from 0.57 for panic disorder to 0.88 for social anxiety disorder.[15] Further, clinician ratings of the clinical utility of the ICD-11 diagnostic guidelines were very positive, indicating that these were easy to use, and corresponded accurately to patients' presentations.[16]

Generalized Anxiety Disorder

ICD-11 GAD has a more elaborated set of essential features than does ICD-10.[19] General apprehensiveness was retained as an alternative to worry in order to ensure cross-cultural applicability and was expanded to include excessive worry about negative events in several different aspects of life. The ICD-11 clinical description of essential features of GAD requires that the general apprehensiveness or worry be accompanied by characteristic symptoms such as muscle tension and sympathetic autonomic overactivity. In the section on additional features, ICD-11 notes that some individuals with GAD may only report chronic somatic anxiety and a feeling of nonspecific dread without being able to articulate specific worry content, and that behavioural changes, such as avoidance and frequent need for reassurance, may be seen.

The ICD-11 diagnostic guidelines for GAD follow the general principles of the clinical descriptions developed for Mental, Behavioural, or Neurodevelopmental Disorders.[20] First, guidance is provided regarding hierarchical exclusion and about clinical significance. Thus, it is emphasized that the GAD symptoms are not better accounted for by another mental disorder (e.g., a depressive disorder), that the symptoms are not a manifestation of another medical condition (e.g., hyperthyroidism) and are not due to the effects of a substance or medication on the central nervous system (e.g., caffeine), including withdrawal effects (e.g., alcohol), and that the symptoms result in significant distress or significant impairment in personal, family, social, educational, occupational, or other important areas of functioning. Whereas ICD-10 did not allow the concurrent diagnosis of GAD and a depressive episode, this is possible in ICD-11 as long as GAD symptoms are not exclusively contiguous with depressive episodes.

Second, pseudo-precise features such as exact symptom duration are avoided; instead, it is noted that symptoms persist for at least several months, for more days than not. Epidemiological data may be useful in investigating proposed changes to diagnostic features,[21] and in support of the ICD-11 approach to the duration of GAD the WHO World Health Mental Surveys (WHMS) found little difference between GAD of 6 months' duration and GAD of shorter durations (1–2 months, 3–5 months) in age of onset, symptom severity or persistence, co-occurrence with other disorders, or impairment.[22] Third, where appropriate, guidance is provided regarding age, gender, and cultural aspects of the clinical descriptions.[23] These principles hold throughout the chapter on Mental, Behavioural, or Neurodevelopmental Disorders, and so will not be repeated for other disorders covered in this chapter.

Panic Disorder

In ICD-11, panic disorder is characterized by recurrent, unexpected panic attacks, which are discrete episodes of intense fear or apprehension with rapid and concurrent onset of several characteristic symptoms.[24] At least some of the panic attacks are unexpected; they are not restricted to particular stimuli or situations but rather seem to arise 'out of the blue'. The focus of apprehension in Panic Disorder is the concern about recurrence of unexpected panic attacks or their significance. In the section on additional features, ICD-11 notes that panic attack length, frequency, and severity vary widely, that some individuals with panic disorder experience nocturnal panic attacks (waking from sleep in a state of panic), and that some individuals present repeatedly for emergency care and may undergo a range of unnecessary special medical investigations.

Panic attacks can occur in the context of other mental disorders and can be indicated using the 'with panic attacks' specifier. Thus, when panic attacks are present in most conditions listed in the Anxiety and Fear-Related Disorders (i.e., generalized anxiety disorder, agoraphobia, social anxiety disorder, specific phobia, and separation anxiety disorder) the specifier 'with panic attacks' can be added. In individuals with panic disorder, panic attacks may become more 'expected' over time as they become associated with particular stimuli or contexts. Limited-symptom panic attacks, in which only a few panic attack symptoms are felt, and without the characteristic intense peak of symptoms, are common in people with panic disorder and may also occur in those with other anxiety disorders.

Agoraphobia

In ICD-11, agoraphobia is conceptualized as marked and excessive fear or anxiety that occurs in, or in anticipation of, multiple situations where escape is difficult or help unavailable.[24] The focus of apprehension is fear of specific negative outcomes occurring in the situations that would be incapacitating or embarrassing. This results in avoidance, or situations may be entered under specific conditions, or endured with intense fear or anxiety. This is a broader construct than that found in ICD-10, which focused on fear of open spaces and related situations, where an escape to a safe place may be difficult. In the section on additional features, ICD-11 notes that individuals with agoraphobia may employ a range of different behavioural strategies to enter feared situations.

In ICD-11, agoraphobia and panic disorder may be diagnosed separately or concurrently (whereas in ICD-10, agoraphobia could be diagnosed as 'with panic disorder' or 'without panic disorder', and a co-occurring diagnosis of both agoraphobia and panic disorder was not permitted). Where individuals with agoraphobia have a history of panic attacks, it may be useful to determine whether an individual's focus of apprehension relates specifically to experiencing symptoms of a panic attack in multiple situations, as this may influence whether components of panic disorder treatment (e.g., interoceptive exposure) are employed, even in the absence of a panic disorder diagnosis.

Specific Phobia
The focus of apprehension in specific phobia is directly connected to encountering or anticipating one or more specific objects or situations (e.g., proximity to certain kinds of animals, heights, enclosed spaces, sight of blood or injury) that is out of proportion to the actual danger posed by the specific object or situation. Active avoidance is not necessary; enduring exposure with intense anxiety is sufficient. In the section on additional features, ICD-11 notes that the most common phobic stimuli include particular animals (animal phobia), heights (acrophobia), enclosed spaces (claustrophobia), sight of blood or injury (blood-injury phobia), and flying. Responses to phobic stimuli can range from feelings of disgust and revulsion, anticipation of danger or harm, and fainting (particularly in response to blood or injury).

Social Anxiety Disorder
Social Anxiety Disorder (SAD) is characterized by marked and excessive fear or anxiety that occurs in social situations, doing something while feeling observed, or performing in front of others. The focus of apprehension is the concern about behaviour that will be negatively evaluated (i.e., that will be humiliating, embarrassing, lead to rejection, or be offensive). Relevant social situations are avoided or endured with intense anxiety. In the section on additional features, ICD-11 notes that individuals with SAD may report concerns about physical symptoms, such as blushing, sweating, or trembling rather than initially voicing fears of negative evaluation, that SAD frequently co-occurs with other anxiety and mood disorders, and that individuals with SAD order are at higher risk for developing substance use disorders (due to self-medication of anxious symptoms).

Separation Anxiety Disorder
In ICD-11, Separation Anxiety Disorder can be diagnosed in adults as well as in children. The focus of apprehension is separation from attachment figures with whom the individual has a deep emotional bond. In children and adolescents, these key attachment figures most commonly include parents, caregivers, and other family members, while in adults they most commonly involve a spouse, romantic partner, or children. Specific manifestations of fear or anxiety related to separation vary according to the individual's developmental level but may include persistent thoughts that harm will lead to separation, recurrent nightmares about separation, and physical symptoms (e.g., nausea, vomiting, stomach ache) on occasions that involve separation from the attachment figure.

Selective Mutism
Selective mutism is characterized by consistent failure to speak in certain situations (e.g., school) despite speaking in other situations (e.g., home). The duration of the disturbance is not transient (e.g., at least several months). The disturbance is not due to a lack of knowledge of, or comfort with, the spoken language demanded in the social situation. In the section on additional features, ICD-11 notes that symptoms may interfere with direct assessment of expressive language, but that children may cooperate with receptive language testing if this is restricted to carrying out commands or pointing to pictures. Selective mutism has been conceptualized as a variant of SAD, given anxious symptoms in social situations, fears of negative evaluation of speech, and anxiety disorder co-morbidity.

Obsessive-Compulsive and Related Disorders

Some obsessive-compulsive and related disorders are characterized by unwanted thoughts or preoccupations, accompanied by rituals and/or other repetitive behaviours. Others are characterized by repetitive motoric behaviours (e.g., tics) or body-focused behaviours (e.g., hair-pulling, skin-picking) without a clear cognitive component. A first step of the ICD-11 Working Group on Obsessive-Compulsive and Related Disorders was to review the literature on these conditions, with a particular focus on clinical utility and global applicability.[8] As noted earlier, the WHO's Global Practice Network was then employed to assess the diagnostic accuracy and clinical utility of proposed ICD-11 diagnostic guidelines for Obsessive-Compulsive and Related Disorders, and these were subsequently revised on the basis of findings from this work.[18]

Obsessive-Compulsive Disorder

Obsessive-compulsive disorder is the central exemplar of the OCRDs and is listed first in the OCRD section.[25] Obsessions are repetitive and persistent thoughts, mental images, or impulses/urges that are experienced as intrusive and unwanted and are commonly associated with anxiety. The individual typically attempts to ignore or suppress obsessions or to neutralize them by performing compulsions. Compulsions are repetitive behaviours or rituals, including repetitive mental acts, that the individual feels driven to perform in response to an obsession, according to rigid rules, or to achieve a sense of 'completeness'. Compulsions either are not connected in a realistic way to the feared event or are clearly excessive.

It is clinically useful to assess degree of insight in individuals with OCD; this can be fair to good or poor to absent. Whereas delusional OCD is relatively rare (less than 4% of cases), it is more common in body dysmorphic disorder (about 30%), and particularly common in ORD (about 70%).[26] Such patients may be less likely to be motivated for treatment, but there is evidence that they may nevertheless respond to first-line treatments for OCD (i.e., SRIs). ICD-10 allowed clinicians to differentiate between OCD with predominantly obsessions and predominantly compulsions, but it has been increasingly recognized that most patients (with the exception of children) have both obsessions and compulsions, and this subtyping is no longer included. There is ongoing research attention to OCD symptom dimensions, but as these do not necessarily impact clinical intervention, they are also not listed as subtypes.

In the section on associated features, ICD notes that individuals with OCD may experience a range of responses when confronted with stimuli that trigger symptoms; these include anxiety or panic attacks, feelings of disgust, or a sense of 'incompleteness' until things are 'just right'. Individuals with OCD may avoid people, places, or things that are such triggers. It is also noteworthy that individuals with OCD may have a range of cognitive distortions, including an inflated sense of responsibility, overestimation of threat, intolerance of uncertainty, and overvaluation of the power of thoughts (e.g., having an aggressive thought is regarded as if one had behaved aggressively).

Body Dysmorphic Disorder

Body dysmorphic disorder (BDD) is characterized by persistent preoccupation with one or more perceived defects or flaws in appearance, or ugliness in general, that are either unnoticeable or only slightly noticeable to others.[14] The individual is excessively self-conscious about the perceived defect or flaw, often including ideas of self-reference, and there is at least one of the following: 1) repeated and excessive behaviours such as repeated examination of the appearance or severity of the perceived defect(s) or flaw(s) or comparison of the relevant feature with that of others, 2) excessive attempts to camouflage or alter the perceived defect, and 3) marked avoidance of social or other situations or stimuli that increase distress about the perceived defect(s) or flaw(s). As with OCD, it is clinically useful to assess degree of insight in individuals with BDD; this can be fair to good or poor to absent.

A range of findings support the inclusion of BDD in the OCRD grouping.[14] The preoccupations and repetitive behaviours are reminiscent of the obsessions and compulsions of OCD, and there is greater than chance co-occurrence between the two disorders. Both OCD and BDD respond to treatment with the serotonergic tricyclic clomipramine, but not to the noradrenergic tricyclic desipramine. Cognitive-behavioural therapy for BDD can be conceptualized as a modification of classic exposure and response prevention for OCD. Nevertheless, it is also important to be aware of crucial distinctions between OCD and BDD with regard to assessment and management; for example, suicide is a particularly important risk in BDD.

The ICD-11 section on additional features notes that any part of the body may be the focus of concern, but the most common area is the face, and there are frequently multiple perceived defects. It is also important to recognize that occurrence of shame and perceived stigma among affected individuals often leads them to conceal their difficulties, making diagnosis difficult. Muscle dysmorphia is a subtype of BDD in which patients have particular concerns about not being sufficiently muscular; this subtype is more common in male patients and is more likely to be associated with the use of steroid agents. In BDD by proxy, individuals are persistently preoccupied with one or more perceived defects or flaws in appearance, or ugliness in general, of another person, that is either unnoticeable or only slightly noticeable to others.

Olfactory Reference Disorder

Olfactory reference disorder (ORD) is characterized by persistent preoccupation about emitting a foul or offensive body odour or breath that is either unnoticeable or slightly noticeable to others such that the individual's concerns are markedly disproportionate to the smell.[14] The individual exhibits excessive self-consciousness about the perceived odour, often including ideas of self-reference, and there is at least one of the following: (1) repetitive and excessive behaviours, such as repeatedly checking for body odour or checking the perceived source of the smell, or repeatedly seeking reassurance by repeated and excessive checking, (2) excessive attempts to camouflage, alter, or prevent the perceived odour, and (3) marked avoidance of social or other situations or stimuli that increase distress about the perceived foul or offensive odour. As with OCD and BDD, it is clinically useful to assess degree of insight in individuals with ORD, which can be specified as fair to good or poor to absent.

Although ORD has not been as well studied as BDD, its symptoms closely parallel those of BDD, with concerns focusing on olfactory rather than visual stimuli. Furthermore, a considerable case report literature suggests that a number of individuals with this condition respond to treatment with serotonin reuptake inhibitors (SRIs). ORD may be misdiagnosed as schizophrenia and treated with high doses of antipsychotics; the inclusion of ORD as an OCRD is clinically useful insofar as it reminds clinicians to consider employing first-line treatments for OCD. At the same time, much further research on ORD is needed to delineate its psychobiology, to assess the extent to which it overlaps with OCD and BDD, and to determine the optimal pharmacotherapy and psychotherapy approach to this condition. Inclusion as a separate category will, it is hoped, advance this research agenda.

Hypochondriasis (Health Anxiety Disorder)

Hypochondriasis (health anxiety disorder) is characterized by persistent preoccupation or fear about the possibility of having one or more serious, progressive, or life-threatening illnesses.[27] This is accompanied by either repetitive and excessive health-related behaviours or maladaptive avoidant behaviours related to health. The health-related behaviours are focused on confirming or disconfirming a medical diagnosis, and may include repeated checking the body for evidence of illness, spending excessive time searching for information about the feared illness, and repeatedly seeking reassurance. In ICD-11, the presence of somatic symptoms is not a required feature and hypochondriasis is no longer classified as a somatoform disorder. As with the other OCRDs, it is clinically useful to assess degree of insight in individuals with hypochondriasis; this can specified as being fair to good or poor to absent.

A range of findings support the inclusion of hypochondriasis in the OCRD grouping.[27] The preoccupations and repetitive behaviours are reminiscent of the obsessions and compulsions of OCD, and there is greater than chance co-morbidity between the two disorders. Both OCD and hypochondriasis respond to treatment with SRIs, and cognitive-behavioural therapy for hypochondriasis can be conceptualized as a modification of that used in OCD. That said, there are also arguments for conceptualizing hypochondriasis as an anxiety disorder,[27] and it is therefore cross-listed among the Anxiety and Fear-Related Disorders. Individuals may have a high level of anxiety about health, be hypervigilant of bodily sensations and symptoms, become easily alarmed about their personal health status, and present with anxiety or panic attacks; hence, 'health anxiety disorder' is included as an alternative name.

The ICD-11 section on additional features notes that individuals with hypochondriasis often make catastrophic misinterpretations of bodily signs or symptoms, including normal or commonplace sensations, and may undergo repeated and unnecessary medical examinations and diagnostic tests, with deterioration of the clinician–patient relationship and frequent 'doctor-shopping'. With increased availability of digital technology, individuals with hypochondriasis may also spend excessive time searching health and medical sites on the internet (cyberchondria). Alternatively, individuals with hypochondriasis may respond to their anxiety about their health by avoiding contact with reminders of health status, including medical check-ups, health facilities, and health-related information. Finally, individuals with hypochondriasis may have increased symptoms when someone they know is sick, when they read or hear about illness, or in response to life stressors.

While the current chapter has not focused primarily on distinctions between ICD-11 and DSM-5, a number of distinctions between ICD-11 hypochondriasis (health anxiety disorder) and DSM-5 illness anxiety disorder are noteworthy.[28] First, ICD-11 hypochondriasis does not exclude individuals with prominent somatic symptoms, whereas in DSM-5 individuals with both illness preoccupations and somatic symptoms are diagnosed with somatic symptom disorder. Second, ICD-11 focuses on fear of having a serious illness, while DSM-5 broadens this to preoccupation with having or acquiring serious illness. Third, ICD-11 specifiers focus on insight, while DSM-5 specifiers focus on care-seeking versus care-avoidance. Fourth, ICD-11 includes a clinical criterion (describing distress and impairment), while DSM-5 does not. Fifth, ICD-11 lists hypochondriasis under OCRDs and Anxiety and Fear-Related Disorders, while DSM-5 lists illness anxiety disorder as a Somatic Symptom and Related Disorder. In our view, given overlap in phenomenology and treatment approaches between hypochondriasis, anxiety, and obsessive-compulsive disorders, the ICD-11 approach has greater clinical utility. However, more sceptical readers may wish to reserve judgement until further research emerges.

Hoarding Disorder

Hoarding disorder is characterized by accumulation of possessions, so that living spaces become cluttered to the point that use or safety is compromised.[29] Accumulation occurs due to repetitive urges or behaviours to amass items as well as due to difficulty discarding them due to a perceived need to save items and distress associated with discarding them. Items are accumulated because of their emotional significance, intrinsic value, or potential usefulness. Similar to the other OCRDs with a cognitive component, it is clinically useful to assess degree of insight in individuals with hoarding disorder, which can be specified as being fair to good or poor to absent. Individuals with hoarding disorder vary in their degree of insight.

A range of findings support the inclusion of hoarding disorder in the OCRD grouping.[29] The phenomenology of hoarding disorder is partly reminiscent of OCD despite the absence of classic compulsions, and there is greater than chance co-occurrence between the two disorders. Cognitive-behavioural therapy for hoarding disorder can be conceptualized as a modification of OCD treatment. On the other hand, there are also important differences between the two conditions; it is notable, for example, that hoarding disorder appears not to respond as robustly as OCD to treatment with SRIs.

The ICD-11 section on additional features notes that individuals with hoarding disorder may be unable to find important items, circulate easily inside their home, or even exit their home in the event of an emergency. Ability to prepare food or use sinks or home appliances or furniture may also be compromised. Individuals with hoarding disorder may experience a range of chronic medical problems, such as obesity, and are exposed to various environmental risks often caused by their hoarding behaviour. Investigations of diagnostic validators of hoarding disorder, as well as of its public health significance, contributed to the decision to include this condition as a new entity in both DSM-5 and ICD-11.[29,30]

Tourette Syndrome

Tourette syndrome is classified primarily as a motoric disorder, and is characterized by the presence of both chronic motor tics and vocal tics.[31] Motor and vocal tics are sudden, rapid, non-rhythmic, and recurrent movements or vocalizations, respectively. Both motor and vocal tics must have been present for at least 1 year, although they may not manifest concurrently or consistently throughout the symptomatic course, with onset during the developmental period. The ICD-11 section on additional features notes that Tourette syndrome frequently occurs with attention deficit hyperactivity disorder, and the two may have overlapping symptoms such as impulsivity. Motor and phonic tics in Tourette syndrome may be voluntarily suppressed for short periods of time, may be exacerbated by stress, and may diminish during sleep or during periods of focused enjoyable activity.

There are several reasons for cross-listing Tourette syndrome in OCRDs.[31] Many patients with OCD have tics, and many patients with Tourette syndrome have OCD.

Further, although repetitive vocal and motor tics in Tourette syndrome appear to be unintentional and are not aimed at neutralizing obsessions, it may be clinically difficult to distinguish the complex tics of Tourette syndrome from the compulsions of OCD. In particular families, some individuals may have Tourette syndrome, whereas others have OCD, and there is ongoing research on the nature of the neurogenetic and neurocircuitry overlap across these conditions. There may also be overlap in the assessment methods and treatment of Tourette syndrome and OCRDs; dopamine antagonists and habit reversal therapy may play a role in a number of these conditions.

Body-Focused Repetitive Behaviour Disorders

The ICD-11 body-focused repetitive behaviour disorders include trichotillomania and excoriation disorder.[32,33] They are characterized by recurrent and habitual actions directed at the integument (e.g., hair pulling, skin picking), typically accompanied by unsuccessful attempts to decrease or stop the behaviour involved, and leading to dermatological sequelae (e.g., hair loss, skin lesions).[34,35] The ICD-11 section on associated features notes that these behaviours may occur in brief episodes scattered throughout the day or in less frequent but more sustained periods, and that the behaviours may be associated with affect and arousal regulation and tension reduction.

Although these conditions share some phenomenological features with the other OCRDs, including ritualistic and repetitive behaviours, they do not have a clear cognitive component. Their psychobiology also shows only partial overlap with other OCRDs; although there is evidence of striatal involvement, this seems less specific than it may be for OCD. Although clomipramine may be more effective than desipramine for trichotillomania, this condition does not demonstrate as robust a response to treatment with SRIs as is seen in OCD. Perhaps a particularly important justification for including these conditions in the OCRDs is to help ensure that more clinicians are aware of them, and to help promote the potential value of screening questions for increasing appropriate diagnosis and treatment.[36,37]

Response to Allen Frances

Allen Frances was critical of some elements in this group of disorders in his Chapter 2 of this volume. Allen is a thoughtful critic and some of his comments are well made. Hoarding disorder shows overlap with other conditions, but this is not a reason for failing to diagnose it, as many other disorders have associated morbidity. The diagnostic criteria make it very clear that it is different from the collecting tendencies of advancing age or the expression of undue nostalgia.

Conclusion

Some seem to have envisaged the psychiatric classification system as a Periodic Table for mental disorders, in which each entity would be clearly demarcated by the provision of necessary and sufficient diagnostic criteria. In this schema, groupings of psychiatric disorder might be similar to the columns or rows of the Periodic Table, carving nature at her joints. However, it is increasingly clear that the nature of mental disorders is simply not like that of the chemical elements, and is instead reminiscent of the more dappled nature of biological entities; psychiatric conditions have fuzzy boundaries from normality and from one another, and they involve a range of causal mechanisms.[38] Furthermore, there is a range of different approaches to delineating the meta-structure of our classification systems, which must aim at being fit for purpose.[39,40]

The ICD-11 arguably takes a conceptual approach that acknowledges this fuzzy nature of mental disorders and that accentuates the strategy that classification systems must be fit for purpose. First, ICD-11 does away with pseudo-specific criteria for mental disorders, so acknowledging the way in which clinicians employ clinical descriptions with clinical judgement. Second, ICD-11 allows dual listing of health conditions, therefore acknowledging that there may be multiple ways of carving up nature. Third, the focus of ICD-11 on clinical utility and global applicability ensures that decisions are weighted less towards neurobiological validators and more towards the issue of practical wisdom in daily clinical work as well as public health considerations.[41,42]

This conceptual approach does not, however, mean that 'anything goes'.[43] Since the publication of DSM-III and ICD-9, considerable nosological research has been undertaken on mental disorders in general, and on anxiety and obsessive-compulsive disorders in particular, and both DSM-5 and ICD-11 are clearly informed by this knowledge.[44] Both classification systems attempted to take a systematic approach to synthesizing research, to being transparent about their decision making, and to gathering new data to inform their final decisions.[13,45] Both classification systems also asked for and responded to a range of feedback from professional bodies and from consumer advocates.[46,47] It is hoped that the two classification systems will, in turn, lead to improved diagnostic practices and so, ultimately, to better clinical interventions around the world.

References

1. Andrews, G., Charney, D.S., Sirovatka, P.J., Regier, D.A. (Eds.) (2009). *Stress-Induced and Fear Circuitry Disorders: Advancing the Research Agenda for DSM-V*. Arlington, VA: American Psychiatric Association.

2. Hollander, E., Zohar, J., Sirovatka. P.J., Regier. D.A. (Eds.) (2011) *Obsessive-Compulsive Spectrum Disorders: Refining the Research Agenda for DSM-V*. Arlington, VA: American Psychiatric Association.

3. Hyman, S.E. (2007). Can neuroscience be integrated into the DSM-V? *Nat Rev Neurosci*, 8(9), 725–732.

4. Regier, D.A., Narrow, W.E., Kuhl, E.A., Kupfer, D.J. (2009). The conceptual development of DSM-V. AJP, **166**(6), 645–850.

5. Kupfer, D.J., Regier, D.A. (2011). Neuroscience, clinical evidence, and the future of psychiatric classification in DSM-5. AJP, **168**(7), 672–674.

6. Kogan, C.S., Stein, D.J., Maj, M., et al. (2016). The classification of anxiety and fear-related disorders in the ICD-11: review: anxiety and fear-related disorders in ICD-11. *Depress Anxiety*, 33(12), 1141–1154.

7. Phillips, K.A., Stein, D.J., Rauch, S.L., et al. (2010). Should an obsessive-compulsive spectrum grouping of disorders be included in DSM-V? *Depress Anxiety*, **27**(6), 528–555.

8. Stein, D.J., Kogan, C.S., Atmaca, M., et al. (2016). The classification of obsessive–compulsive and related disorders in the ICD-11. *J Affect Disord*, 190, 663–874.

9. Stein, D.J., Fineberg, N.A., Bienvenu, O.J., et al. (2010). Should OCD be classified as an anxiety disorder in DSM-V? *Depress Anxiety*, 27(6), 495–506.

10. Phillips, K.A., Friedman, M.J., Stein, D.J., Craske, M. (2010). Special DSM-V issues on anxiety, obsessive-compulsive spectrum, posttraumatic, and dissociative disorders. *Depress Anxiety*, 27(2), 91–92.

11. Stein, D.J., Craske, M.A., Friedman, M.J., Phillips, K.A. (2014). Anxiety disorders, obsessive-compulsive and related

disorders, trauma- and stressor-related disorders, and dissociative disorders in DSM-5. *AJP*, **171**(6), 611–613.

12. Keeley, J.W., Reed, G.M., Roberts, M.C., et al. (2016). Developing a science of clinical utility in diagnostic classification systems: field study strategies for ICD-11 mental and behavioral disorders. *Am Psychol*, **71**(1), 3–16.

13. Stein, D.J., Szatmari, P., Gaebel, W., et al. (2020). Mental, behavioral and neurodevelopmental disorders in the ICD-11: an international perspective on key changes and controversies. *BMC Med*, **18**(1), 21.

14. Veale, D., Matsunaga, H. (2014). Body dysmorphic disorder and olfactory reference disorder: proposals for ICD-11. *Braz J Psychiatry*, **36**(suppl 1), 14–20.

15. Reed, G.M., Sharan, P., Rebello, T.J., et al. (2018). The ICD-11 developmental field study of reliability of diagnoses of high-burden mental disorders: results among adult patients in mental health settings of 13 countries. *World Psychiatry*, **17**(2), 174–186.

16. Reed, G.M., Keeley, J.W., Rebello, T.J., et al. (2018). Clinical utility of ICD-11 diagnostic guidelines for high-burden mental disorders: results from mental health settings in 13 countries: clinical utility of ICD-11 diagnostic guidelines for high-burden mental disorders: results from mental health settings in 13 countries. *World Psychiatry*, **17**(3), 306–315.

17. Rebello, T.J., Keeley, J.W., Kogan, C.S., et al. (2019). Anxiety and fear-related disorders in the ICD-11: Results from a global case-controlled field study. *Arch Med Res*, **50**(8), 490–501.

18. Kogan, C.S., Stein, D.J., Rebello, T.J., et al. (2020). Accuracy of diagnostic judgments using ICD-11 vs. ICD-10 diagnostic guidelines for obsessive-compulsive and related disorders. *J Affect Disord*, **273**, 328–340.

19. Shear, K.M. (2012). Generalized anxiety disorder in ICD-11. *World Psychiatry*, **11**(S1), 82–88.

20. First, M.B., Reed, G.M., Hyman, S.E., Saxena, S. (2015). The development of the ICD-11 clinical descriptions and diagnostic guidelines for mental and behavioural disorders. *World Psychiatry*, **14**(1), 82–90.

21. Stein, D.J., Scott, K.M., de Jonge, P., Kessler, R.C. (2017). Epidemiology of anxiety disorders: from surveys to nosology and back. *Dialogues Clin Neurosci*, **19**(2), 127–136.

22. Lee, S., Tsang, A., Ruscio, A.M., et al. (2009). Implications of modifying the duration requirement of generalized anxiety disorder in developed and developing countries. *Psychol Med*, **39**(07), 1163.

23. Gureje, O., Lewis-Fernandez, R., Hall, B.J., Reed, G.M. (2020). Cultural considerations in the classification of mental disorders: why and how in ICD-11. *BMC Med*, **18**(1), 25.

24. Stein, D.J. (2012). Agoraphobia and panic disorder: options for ICD-11. *World Psychiatry*, **11**(suppl 1), 89–93.

25. Simpson, H.B., Reddy, Y.C.J. (2014). Obsessive-compulsive disorder for ICD-11: proposed changes to the diagnostic guidelines and specifiers. *Braz J Psychiatry*, **36**(suppl 1), 3–13.

26. Phillips, K.A., Hart, A.S., Simpson, H.B., Stein, D.J. (2014). Delusional versus nondelusional body dysmorphic disorder: recommendations for DSM-5. *CNS Spectr*, **19**(1), 10–20.

27. van den Heuvel, O.A., Veale, D., Stein, D.J. (2014). Hypochondriasis: considerations for ICD-11. *Braz J Psychiatry*, **36**(suppl 1), 21–27.

28. Phillips, K.A., Rodriguez, C.I., Harding, K.J., Fallon, B.A., Stein, D.J. (2022). Obsessive-compulsive or related disorders: hypochondriasis, hoarding disorder, body dysmorphic disorder, olfactory reference disorder, trichotillomania, and excoriation disorder. In Tasman, A., Riba, M.B., Alarcon, R.D., et al. (Eds.), *Tasman's Psychiatry*, 5th ed. Springer.

29. Fontenelle, L.F., Grant, J.E. (2014). Hoarding disorder: a new diagnostic

30. Mataix-Cols, D., Frost, R.O., Pertusa, A., et al. (2010). Hoarding disorder: a new diagnosis for DSM-V? *Depress Anxiety*, **27**(6), 556–572.

31. Woods, D.W., Thomsen, P.H. (2014). Tourette and tic disorders in ICD-11: standing at the diagnostic crossroads. *Braz J Psychiatry*, **36**(suppl 1), 51–68.

32. Grant, J.E., Stein, D.J. (2014). Body-focused repetitive behavior disorders in ICD-11. *Braz J Psychiatry*, **36**(suppl 1), 59–64.

33. Stein, D.J., Woods, D.W. (2014). Stereotyped movement disorder in ICD-11. *Braz J Psychiatry*, **36**(suppl 1), 65–68.

34. Lochner, C., Grant, J.E., Odlaug, B.L., Stein, D.J. (2012). DSM-5 field survey: skin picking disorder. *Ann Clin Psychiatry*, **24**(4), 300–304.

35. Lochner, C., Grant, J.E., Odlaug, B.L., et al. (2012). DSM-5 field survey: hair-pulling disorder (trichotillomania). *Depress Anxiety*, **29**(12), 1025–1031.

36. Stein, D.J., Grant, J.E., Franklin, M.E., et al. (2010). Trichotillomania (hair pulling disorder), skin picking disorder, and stereotypic movement disorder: toward DSM-V. *Depress Anxiety*, **27**(6), 611–626.

37. Grant, J.E., Odlaug, B.L., Chamberlain, S.R., et al. (2012). Skin picking disorder. *Am J Psychiatry*, **169**(11), 1143–1149.

38. Stein, D. (2021). *Problems of Living: Perspectives from Philosophy, Psychiatry and Cognitive-Affective Science*. Academic Press.

39. Stein, D.J. (2008). Is disorder X in category or spectrum Y? General considerations and application to the relationship between obsessive-compulsive disorder and anxiety disorders. *Depress Anxiety*, **25**, 330–335.

40. Roberts, M.C., Reed, G.M., Medina-Mora, M.E., et al. (2012). A global clinicians' map of mental disorders to improve ICD-11: analysing meta-structure to enhance clinical utility. *Int Rev Psychiatry*, **24**(6), 578–590.

41. Stein, D.J., Reed, G.M. (2019). Global mental health and psychiatric nosology: DSM-5, ICD-11, and RDoC. *Braz J Psychiatry*, **41**(1), 3–4.

42. Stein, D.J., Billieux, J., Bowden-Jones, H., et al. (2018). Balancing validity, utility, and public health considerations in disorders due to addictive behaviors. *World Psychiatry*, 17, 363–364.

43. Feyerabend, P. (1975). *Against Method: Outline of an Anarchistic Theory of Knowledge*. New Left Books.

44. Stein, D.J., Reed, G.M. (2019). ICD-11: the importance of a science of psychiatric nosology. *Lancet Psychiatry*, **6**(1), 6–7.

45. Kendler, K.S. (2013). A history of the DSM-5 scientific review committee. *Psychol Med*, **43**(9), 1793–800.

46. Stein, D.J., Phillips, K.A. (2013). Patient advocacy and DSM-5. *BMC Med*, **11**(1), 133.

47. Fuss, J., Lemay, K., Stein, D.J., et al. (2019). Public stakeholders' comments on ICD-11 chapters related to mental and sexual health. *World Psychiatry*, **18**(2), 233–235.

Chapter 9

Personality Disorders

Roger Mulder

Introduction

When the ICD-11 working group for the revision of the classification of personality disorders was established in 2010, there was both an increasing concern, followed by general consensus, that the existing classifications in ICD-10 and DSM-IV were no longer fit for purpose. First, the system was complex, with around 80 criteria and 10 separate categories. These categories had evolved from historical precedents, clinical experience, and committee consensus. There was no coherent model or theory for the diagnoses. Some categories had their origins in Galen's temperaments described over 1,800 years ago, while others, such as borderline personality disorder, had appeared very recently. Clinicians responded to this confusion by often ignoring the whole concept of personality disorders, resulting in low rates of diagnosis in clinical practice. Rates of clinical diagnoses are generally reported to be less than one-quarter of those in systematic prevalence studies.[1] When clinicians did make a personality disorder diagnosis, they usually confined themselves to 2 of the 10 categories: borderline personality disorder or antisocial personality disorder, or used the catch-all 'personality disorder not otherwise specified' (PD-NOS), or mixed and other personality disorders (61.0) in ICD-10.[2] The complexity of personality disorder nosology meant that interest was confined to a specialist few, with the general clinician feeling out of their depth.

Second, all the evidence pointed towards personality abnormality being distributed along a dimension.[3] There was also evidence that these dimensions were related to the facets of personality reported in the general population, especially the five factor model that has become known as the Big Five.[4] Not surprisingly, normal and abnormal personalities are, at least to some extent, related to each other.[5] There is empirical support for using a dimensional model of personality to understand personality disorders. Four meta-analyses using a total of 13,640 individuals in 52 samples concluded that personality pathology can be adequately represented as constellations of extreme scores on normal personality models, notably the five factor model.[6] It is notable that a number of authors had previously suggested a dimensional approach to the diagnosis of personality disorders,[7,8] but this approach has been slow to be accepted.

Third, there is consistent evidence that the severity rather than the type of personality pathology is the major predictor of the individual's suffering of dysfunction.[9] The total number of personality disorder symptoms explains more variability in functioning than specific personality disorder symptoms.[10] More severe personality disturbance is associated with more self-harm,[11] suicide risk,[12] and psychosocial impairment.[13]

The ICD-11 Classification System

Given this evidence, it is hardly surprising that the ICD-11 working group for the revision of the classification of personality disorders felt a paradigm shift was necessary when they first met in 2010. Tinkering around the edges would not address the fundamental problems with the ICD-10 classification system. Led by Peter Tyrer, the following goals were conceptualized:

- Establish the primacy of severity in measuring personality disorders.
- Eliminate the arbitrary diagnostic thresholds that create the appearance of strict category boundaries.
- Reduce diagnostic co-occurrence among personality categories.
- Reduce heterogeneity of personality categories.
- Eliminate the excessive use of personality disorders not otherwise specified (PDNOS) and mixed disorders.
- Try to implement an empirically based model of personality disorder structure that is consistent with the structure of personality in the general population.

Severity

To achieve these goals, the initial proposal for ICD-11 classification set out to abolish all (type-specific) categories of personality disorder apart from the general description of a personality disorder. This description was conceptualized along a dimension of severity. Therefore, to qualify for a diagnosis of a personality disorder, there were general diagnostic features such as problems with functioning of aspects of the self and/or interpersonal dysfunction manifest in various patterns of emotional expression and maladaptive behaviour across a range of situations (see WHO (2018)[14] for a full definition). The diagnosis could then be further specified as 'mild', 'moderate', or 'severe' based on descriptions of degrees of severity. Assessment of severity is based on the prominence of abnormal traits and their impact on the individual's social and occupational functioning, as well as the risk they pose to themselves or others. Mild personality disorder affects some areas of personality functioning in some contexts and is not associated with substantial harm to others. Moderate personality disorder affects multiple areas of personality functioning with marked problems in most interpersonal relationships and may be associated with harm to self or others. Severe personality disorder manifests as severe disturbance in self and interpersonal functioning, affects all relationships, and is often associated with harm to self and others (see WHO (2018)[14] for a full definition).

Personality Difficulty

'Personality difficulty' is a new term in ICD-11 and is related to severity. It is a subsyndromal diagnosis related to 'problems associated with interpersonal interactions'. More specifically, the definition refers to 'pronounced personality characteristics that may affect treatment or health services but do not rise to the level of severity to merit a diagnosis of personality disorder'.[14] In contrast to personality disorders, personality difficulty is manifest in 'cognitive and emotional experience and expression only intermittently (e.g. during times of stress) or at low intensity'.[14] However, while not a diagnosis, this does not mean it can be ignored. The differences between personality difficulty and disorder are shown in Table 9.1.

Table 9.1 Differences between personality difficulty and personality disorder

Personality difficulty	Personality disorder
Intermittent presentation	Persistent presentation
Confined to certain situations	Present in all situations
Does not interfere greatly with normal social and occupational performance	Impairs social and occupational performance
Not associated with risk of harm to self or others	Often associated with risk of harm to self or others

Because personality difficulty is remarkably common it should not be ignored. It has an influence on the outcome of other mental disorders, and may change into a formal personality disorder (or vice versa).[15] As one example, Yang et al.[16] defined personality difficulty as a score of one operational criterion less than a personality disorder on the UK National Morbidity Survey ($n = 8,400$) and reported a high prevalence of 48.3 per cent. These individuals were more likely to consult their GP, be admitted to a psychiatric hospital, attend a community medical centre, or see a mental health worker, so it cannot be regarded as a trivial addition to the system.[16]

There are concerns that the term will lead to over-medicalization of difficult behaviour and become reified as a diagnosis, even though it is explicitly stated it is not one. If there is distress or greater help-seeking at any level of diagnosis, this justifies its description. The term may also help in understanding the concept of a personality spectrum and reduce stigma when it is realized that it is present in a significant proportion of the population. and probably more common than those with no personality problems.

Personality Trait Domain Qualifiers

Although the concept of a dimension of personality pathology was a major change in classification, it fitted in with most clinicians' and researchers' views of the evidence. A similar proposal was put forward for DSM-5. A conscious decision was made to separate the two issues of 'disorder' and 'behavioural manifestations' by the DSM committee. But how to describe these behavioural manifestations was more controversial. Among clinicians with a special interest in personality disorders, there was considerable belief that individual categories such as narcissistic, borderline, and antisocial had clinical meaning and could not be linked to dimensional variation.

The ICD-11 working group felt that as the evidence supported a single spectrum of personality disturbance, to include the arbitrary ICD-10 categories was of no value and these should be abandoned. However, it was also clear that clinicians needed ways to describe personality pathology. The change envisaged was hardly novel. There was strong consensus that ICD-10 and DSM-IV categories were unsatisfactory and should be replaced.[3] The main problem was that there was no consistency on what should be used to replace them.[1]

There were some practical constraints; the description of behavioural disturbance needed to be useful in all medical settings in all countries, including low- and middle-income ones; it needed to be reasonably simple and concise as well as clinically useful. We wished it to be as evidence-based as possible and to link personality disorder descriptions with 'normal' personality in community samples if the evidence supported this.

Empirical Foundation of Trait Domain Qualifiers

The ICD-11 proposal was guided by a systematic review of the personality disorder literature which identified 1,408 studies potentially studying the empirical domains of personality disorders.[1] Despite using different patient samples, different models of personality pathology, various means to assess personality, and subjecting the findings to multiple statistical manipulations, the results were surprisingly consistent. All studies reported a general 'personality pathology' dimension as predicted but also an externalizing and internalizing domain. Most reported a schizoid/aloof domain, and the majority, a compulsivity domain.

Although these four factors were reported reasonably consistently across studies and had good face validity, the externalizing domain encompassed a wide range of behaviours including antisocial, psychopathy, and impulsivity. After much debate, a factor incorporating non-psychopathic externalizing behaviours – disinhibition – was introduced for further study. The ICD-11 therefore consists of five broad descriptions of personality pathology called trait domain qualifiers. It is important to note that they are not categories but descriptive domains used 'to describe the characteristics of the individual's personality that are most prominent and that contribute to personality disturbance'.[14] As many trait domain qualifiers as necessary may be applied to describe personality functioning. Individuals with more severe personality disturbance tend to have greater numbers of prominent trait domains.

Brief Description of Trait Domain Qualifiers

- Negative Affectivity – a tendency to experience a broad range of negative emotions with a frequency and intensity out of proportion to the situation, which may include emotional lability, negative attitudes, and low self-esteem
- Dissociality – a disregard for the rights and feelings of others, encompassing both self-centeredness and lack of empathy
- Detachment – a tendency to maintain interpersonal and emotional detachment from others
- Disinhibition – a tendency to act rashly based on immediate external and internal stimuli without consideration of potential negative consequences
- Anankastia – a tendency towards perfectionism and orderliness and emotional and behavioural constraint

(See WHO, 2018[14] for full descriptions.)

Measuring the ICD-11 Trait Domains

One problem with a radical change in a classification system is that the findings or previous studies cannot be directly translated into the new system. The ICD-11 classification is not accompanied by a measure that provides a formal operationalization of the classification system.[17] Initial attempts to validate the ICD-11 system used DSM-IV symptoms to represent the trait domains. Kim et al. (2015)[18] reported that the anankastic, detached, and dissocial domains were coherent and discriminated well, but the emotionally unstable and anxious/dependent (as they were then called) were less robust. Mulder et al. (2016)[19] found that the best-fitting model comprised five domains, with anankastia, detached, and dissocial closely matching the ICD-11 proposal. The negative affectivity and disinhibition domains were less distinctly represented, but it should be noted that few of the relevant terms for these domains are in the DSM-IV classification.

Bach and colleagues noted that the ICD-11 and DSM-5 Alternative Model for Personality Disorders (AMPD) (the system adopted after the original classification was rejected by the American Psychiatric Association) shared four of the five domains, the only exception being anankastia in the ICD-11 model versus psychoticism in the AMPD. This allowed them to translate the extensive research on the AMPD trait domains into the ICD-11 domain traits. Bach et al. (2017)[20] developed an algorithm for delineating all five ICD-11 trait domains (including a separate domain of anankastia) by means of the well-established personality inventory for DSM-5 (PID-5[21]). They showed that 16 PID-5 facets could generate the five ICD-11 domain scores and that the five factor structure was validated across US and Danish samples.[20] Since then, a number of studies have validated the ICD-11 algorithm for PID-5 in different populations[22] including an Iranian sample[23] and a Brazilian sample.[24] Sellbom et al.[25] further improved the ICD-11 algorithm by including two more PID-5 facets (suspiciousness and attention-seeking). The empirical structure was supported in a sample of Canadian psychiatric patients and, in addition, demonstrated expected associations with categorical personality disorder criterion-count scores, similar to those reported by Bach et al. (2018) (Table 9.2).[22]

By 2018, Oltmanns and Widiger had introduced the first instrument specifically developed for the ICD-11 trait domains – the Personality Inventory for ICD-11 (PiCD).[26] The PiCD consists of 60 items used to calculate the five ICD-11 domain scores (i.e., 12 items per domain). The PiCD has been evaluated in a number of studies supporting the validity of the trait domains.[27] Importantly, the ICD-11 trait domains also showed meaningful and expected relationships with normal personality dimensions measured using Eysenck's trait model and the five factor model. Negative affectivity corelated with neuroticism, detachment with low extraversion, dissociality with insensitivity, anankastia with high orderliness, and disinhibition with low orderliness.[28] Oltmanns and Widiger (2020)[29] have gone on to develop a 121-item Five Factor Personality Inventory for ICD-11 which provides facet-level operationalization of the ICD-11 trait domains.

Given the similarity between the ICD-11 and DSM-5 AMPD trait domain personality measures, Kerber et al. (2020)[30] proposed a 34-item Personality Inventory for DSM-5, Brief Form Plus (PID5BF+), which aims to capture both DSM-5 and ICD-11 trait domains and which includes anankastia and psychoticism. This measure has demonstrated good scale reliability and expected discriminant and criterion validity. Bach et al. (2020)[31] modified this measure, which now comprises 36 items that measure 18 facets and appears robust across different population samples.

The Anankastia Domain Qualifier

This trait domain has been discussed more than the other domains for two reasons: 1) It is not a domain in what is called the Alternative Model for Personality Disorders (AMPD) in DSM-5. 2) Some studies suggest that it is not a separate domain but instead part of a bipolar disinhibition–anankastia factor. Regarding the first reason, compulsivity, which is roughly equal to anankastia, was originally proposed as a distinct domain in the DSM-5 trait model.[32] It was abandoned for reasons which are not clear but which are

Table 9.2 Bivariate associations of ICD-11 personality trait domains with personality disorder criterion count

SCID-II rated personality disorders

	Cluster A			Cluster B				Cluster C		
	PAR	SCD	STY	ANT	BOR	HIS	NAR	AVO	DPT	OBS
Negative Affectivity	**0.45**	0.06	0.33	−0.09	**0.51**	**0.29**	0.05	**0.54**	**0.46**	**0.23**
Detachment	**0.43**	**0.46**	**0.41**	0.26	0.38	0.04	0.23	0.33	0.17	0.15
Dissociality	**0.52**	0.31	0.36	**0.60**	0.43	**0.32**	**0.71**	0.00	0.06	0.26
Disinhibition	0.47	0.28	0.44	**0.49**	**0.60**	**0.43**	0.45	0.18	0.34	0.13
Anankastia	0.44	0.22	0.40	0.15	0.48	0.34	0.25	0.35	0.24	**0.62**

Boldfaced correlations indicate the hypothesized trait domains for each personality disorder type.
Reproduced from the *Australian and New Zealand Journal of Psychiatry* (vol, 52) with permission

probably related to the five factor model. The generated list of 37 facets for the DSM-5 AMPD included (lack of) orderliness, (lack of) perfectionism, and (lack of) rigidity, which are aligned with an anankastic or compulsivity domain. However, these facets were subsumed into the disinhibited domain.[21] Our review[1] found that anankastia, or something very similar, was reported in most analyses which looked for it, while a disinhibition dimension was less consistently found.

That said, there are legitimate concerns about the relationship of the disinhibited and anankastia domains in the ICD-11 classification. Two studies have reported a four factor solution including a bipolar disinhibition–anankastia domain.[26,28] However, other studies support a five factor solution in which anankastia and disinhibition are two distinct domains.[19,20,25] The clinical reality may be that complex personality disorder patterns can be characterized by both disinhibition and anankastia,[33] and the notion that they are polar opposites remains contentious. It is perfectly possible for an individual to score highly for disinhibition and compulsivity and this cannot possibly be accommodated by the Big Five system.

What About Borderline Personality Disorder?

Borderline personality disorder poses a particular problem. On the one hand, it is the most studied personality disorder particularly in relation to treatment. It is also by far the most used diagnosis by clinicians who work in personality disorder treatment settings. However, the evidence base for the treatment of borderline personality disorder essentially tells us that a host of treatments are similarly effective and none has shown specific efficacy for borderline personality disorder as opposed to general psychological distress and dysfunction.[34] In addition, borderline personality disorder does not sit comfortably within personality trait dimensions, and its features are largely clinical symptoms rather than personality traits.[35] Factor analytical studies over the past 20 years have failed to support a distinct borderline personality disorder category.[36] There is increasing evidence that the category is a measure of general impairment in personality functioning and is strongly associated with the overall severity of personality pathology.[37] Within the ICD-11 domains, it is strongly related to negative affectivity and disinhibition, and moderately related to dissociality.

Despite this evidence, letting borderline personality disorder go proved challenging to clinicians specializing in the treatment of personality disorders. They pointed out that losing the diagnosis would have substantial effects on research funding and treatment provision.[38] A pragmatic solution to these objections was reached, allowing clinicians to specify a 'borderline pattern qualifier' (note, not a diagnosis). This essentially consists of the nine DSM-5 borderline diagnostic criteria. Nevertheless, the ICD-11 working group felt that the severity and domain trait model could fully account for the borderline pattern without the need for another diagnostic element.[39]

Implications for Treatment: Clinical Utility

On the face of it, the ICD-11 classification model seems more 'true' to existing evidence about personality pathology. As we have noted, the classification has been operationalized and appears to have robust construct validity and predictable convergence with other personality measures, and demonstrates reliability cross-culturally. However, while construct validity is an essential requirement, it is not sufficient.[34] The most important consequence of a paradigm shift in diagnostic models is to aid the development and evaluation of treatments. A number of frameworks have been proposed which suggest careful assessment of severity and trait domains can lead to a coherent and holistic formulation that can be shared with the patient and a consensual approach to treatment adopted.[27,34]

The general dimension of personality severity may be a good target for intervention and monitoring efficacy and a better way of measuring progress than specific personality features which are more stable.[27,40] Clinicians appear to value the level of personality function more than specific personality disorder categories when formulating treatments and discussing them with patients.[41,42] Severity is also associated with treatment alliance and risk of drop-out[43] as well as boundary confusion and increased negative counter-transference.[44]

Similarly, assessment of domain traits encourages a collaborative therapeutic approach: helping patients identify their own traits and how they are demonstrated in everyday life and conveying the idea that traits can be changed into something more adaptive.[45] Acknowledging the adaptive significance of traits when the context is considered may be important. For example, a patient with detachment may be less emotionally responsive, which is problematic in some social situations but may be useful when cool-headed, self-absorbed behaviour is called for. The therapeutic task may be to measure emotional activity while accepting their detached nature. The general aim of treatment is not to transform individual trait domains but to encourage adaptation and, to some degree, acceptance.

The obvious outstanding problem, of course, is that there are currently no treatment studies using the ICD-11 classification. The clinical utility of severity has considerable general evidence but there are no specific studies utilizing ICD-11 or DSM-5 AMPD, for that matter. Because treatment studies have focused so intensively on borderline personality disorder, there is virtually no evidence for the utility of trait domains, particularly detachment and anankastia, which are less related to borderline personality disorder symptoms.

Tracy et al.[17] have recently completed a preliminary scoping review of the clinical utility of the ICD-11 classification of personality disorders. They concluded that while findings were mixed, in general clinicians felt ICD-11 improved communication between clinicians and had clinical utility, but there were concerns about implementation and feasibility in clinical practice. This may partially reflect how new the model is and its applicability cross-culturally.[17]

What of the Future?

A potential problem is the retention of the borderline pattern descriptor, which may lead clinicians to continue with the current practice of using the borderline pattern and possibly the dissocial trait domain while largely ignoring the other domains. (It should be noted that if the AMPD model were to be adopted, the situation may be worse since they have retained six individual personality disorders.) New research and planning of services would need to change. Instead of simply focusing on borderline personality disorder, most of whose sufferers are likely to have moderate personality disorder with a mix of negative affectivity, disinhibited, and dissocial domain traits, clinicians can now dissect the relevant traits and adjust treatment accordingly. At the very least they will test whether the current borderline heterogeneous grouping can be carefully dissected into more homogeneous traits.[46] In addition, some clinical attention might be focused on those suffering from moderate detachment or anankastia.

We also recommend moving personality disorder diagnosis outside of speciality personality disorder services and mental health services and encourage all health professionals to make an ICD-11 diagnosis in their patients. We know individuals with personality disorder are more likely to consult health professionals than other people at all levels of pathology.[16] We also know that personality disorder status affects treatment acceptance and outcome of both mental and physical illness.[47] We are not advocating a full diagnostic assessment but some attempt to describe prominent personality features that are likely to affect clinical practice. It is likely something most clinicians do subliminally, but it might be better if this understanding was integrated into training.

The average clinician reading this chapter may be somewhat taken aback by the considerable changes in the ICD-11 revision and what it means for their clinical practice. The implications are shown in Table 9.3.

In many countries, there is a change taking place in funding arrangements for mental health, from funding on general service activity towards diagnostic related groups. This is likely to extend to personality disorder, and will need to be recognized in practice, as it is known that personality dysfunction has such impact on service usage.

The likely prevalence of each level of personality dysfunction (Table 9.3) shows that it is impractical to consider specific interventions for personality difficulty. But by highlighting the presence of personality difficulty in the presence of other disorders, a variant of Galenic syndromes, or combined personality and mental state disorders,[48] it should be possible to fashion treatments that address both elements of the combination. To take one specific example, a small number of patients make an excellent clinical response to monoamine oxidase inhibitors such as phenelzine after all other medication has failed.[48] Because of the potential dangers of food interactions with these drugs, it would be unwise to prescribe these

Table 9.3 Likely prevalence of personality dysfunction using ICD-11 criteria and possible range of treatments

ICD-10 comparison	ICD-11 diagnosis	Likely prevalence In population	Possible interventions
No equivalent	Personality difficulty	40%	May influence choice of treatments for co-morbid disorders
ICD-10 personality disorder	Mild personality disorder	15%	Matching physical, social, and personal environments to get a better fit
Categories: emotionally unstable, dependent, anxious, dissocial, histrionic, schizoid, paranoid, anankastic	Moderate personality disorder	5%	Specific interventions depending on trait domain mix
	Severe personality disorder	<0.5%	Intensive interventions, often in institutional care

drugs liberally. However, those who are very diligent about taking their medication, and have anankastic personality difficulty, can be relied upon to follow food restrictions carefully. This may extend to more severe personality problems too.[49]

Summary

It might be expected that the authors of a new classification system would promote it strongly, so any praise could be discounted. But all the evidence to date suggests the ICD-11 personality disorder construct is preferred by clinicians, is understood by patients, and is an aid to the selection of treatment. It takes into account the high prevalence of personality disorder in mental health services and should be a spur to better and more sophisticated management. It offers excellent prospects for the future.

References

1. Mulder, R.T., Newton-Howes, G., Crawford, M.J., Tyrer, P.J. (2011). The central domains of personality pathology in psychiatric patients. *J Pers Disord*, **25**(3), 364–377.

2. Verheul, R., Widiger, T.A. (2004). A meta-analysis of the prevalence and usage of the personality disorder not otherwise specified (PDNOS) diagnosis. *J Pers Disord*, **18**(4), 309–319.

3. Bernstein, D.P., Iscan, C., Maser, J., Board of Directors of the Association for Research in Personality Disorders, Board of Directors of the International Society for the Study of Personality Disorders. (2007). Opinions of personality disorder experts regarding the DSM-IV personality disorders classification system. *J Pers Disord*, **21**(5), 536–551.

4. Costa, P.T., McCrae, R.R. (1992). The five-factor model of personality and its relevance to personality disorders. *J Pers Disord*, **6**, 343–359.

5. Hengartner, M.P., Müller, M., Rodgers, S., Rössler, W., Ajdacic-Gross, V. (2014). Interpersonal functioning deficits in association with DSM-IV personality disorder dimensions. *Soc Psychiatry Psychiatr Epidemiol*, **49**(2), 317–325.

6. Gotzsche-Astrup, O., Moskowitz, A. (2016). Personality disorders and the DSM-5: scientific and extra-scientific factors in the maintenance of the status quo. *Aust N Z J Psychiatry*, **50**(2), 119–127.

7. Frances, A. (1982). Categorical and dimensional systems of personality diagnosis: a comparison. *Compr Psychiatry*, **23**(6), 516–527.

8. Ekselius, L., Lindström, E., von Knorring, L., Bodlund, O., Kullgren, G. (1994). A principal component analysis of the DSM-III-R axis II personality disorders. *J Pers Disord*, **8**(2), 140–148.

9. Crawford, M.J., Koldobsky, N., Mulder, R.T., Tyrer, P. (2011). Classifying personality disorder according to severity. *J Pers Disord*, **25**(3), 321–330.

10. Kvarstein, E.H., Karterud, S. (2013). Large variation of severity and longitudinal change of symptom distress among patients with personality disorders. *Personal Ment Health*, **7**(4), 265–276.

11. Blasco-Fontecilla, H., Baca-Garcia, E., Dervic, K., et al. (2009). Severity of personality disorders and suicide attempt. *Acta Psychiatr Scand*, **119**(2), 149–155.

12. Conway, C.C., Hammen, C., Brennan, P.A. (2016). Optimizing prediction of psychosocial and clinical outcomes with a transdiagnostic model of personality disorder. *J Pers Disord*, **30**(4), 545–566.

13. Wright, A.G.C., Hopwood, C.J., Skodol, A.E., Morey, L.C. (2016). Longitudinal validation of general and specific structural features of personality pathology. *J Abnorm Psychol*, **125**(8), 1120–1134.

14. World Health Organization. (2018). *ICD-11, the 11th Revision of the International Classification of Diseases*. Geneva: World

Health Organization. [Available from: https://icd.who.int/.]
15. Yang, M., Tyrer, H., Johnson, T., Tyrer, P. (2021). Personality change in the Nottingham Study of Neurotic Disorder: 30-Year cohort study. *Aust NZ J Psychiatry*, **56**(3), 260–269.
16. Yang, M., Coid, J., Tyrer, P. (2010). Personality pathology recorded by severity: national survey. *Br J Psychiatry*, **197**(3), 193–199.
17. Tracy, M., Tiliopoulos, N., Sharpe, L., Bach, B. (2021). The clinical utility of the ICD-11 classification of personality disorders and related traits: a preliminary scoping review. *Aust NZ J Psychiatry*, **55**(9), 849–862.
18. Kim, Y.-R., Tyrer, P., Lee, H.-S., et al. (2015). Preliminary field trial of a putative research algorithm for diagnosing ICD-11 personality disorders in psychiatric patients: 2. *Proposed trait domains. Personal Ment Health*, **9**(4), 298–307.
19. Mulder, R.T., Horwood, J., Tyrer, P., Carter, J., Joyce, P.R. (2016). Validating the proposed ICD-11 domains. *Personal Ment Health*, **10**(2), 84–95.
20. Bach, B., Sellbom, M., Kongerslev, M., et al. (2017). Deriving ICD-11 personality disorder domains from DSM-5 traits: initial attempt to harmonize two diagnostic systems. *Acta Psychiatr Scand*, **136**(1), 108–117.
21. Krueger, R.F., Derringer, J., Markon, K.E., Watson, D., Skodol, A.E. (2012). Initial construction of a maladaptive personality trait model and inventory for DSM-5. *Psychol Med*, **42**(9), 1879–1890.
22. Bach, B., Sellbom, M., Skjernov, M., Simonsen, E. (2018). ICD-11 and DSM-5 personality trait domains capture categorical personality disorders: finding a common ground. *Aust NZ J Psychiatry*, **52**(5), 425–434.
23. Lotfi, M., Bach, B., Amini, M., Simonsen, E. (2018). Structure of DSM-5 and ICD-11 personality domains in Iranian community sample. *Personal Ment Health*, **12**(2), 155–169.

24. Lugo, V., de Oliveira, S.E.S., Hessel, C.R., et al. (2019). Evaluation of DSM-5 and ICD-11 personality traits using the Personality Inventory for DSM-5 (PID-5) in a Brazilian sample of psychiatric inpatients. *Personal Ment Health*, **13**(1), 24–39.
25. Sellbom, M., Solomon-Krakus, S., Bach, B., Bagby, R.M. (2020). Validation of Personality Inventory for DSM–5 (PID-5) algorithms to assess ICD-11 personality trait domains in a psychiatric sample. *Psychol Assess*, **32**(1), 40–49.
26. Oltmanns, J.R., Widiger, T.A. (2018). A self-report measure for the ICD-11 dimensional trait model proposal: the personality inventory for ICD-11. *Psychol Assess*, **30**(2), 154–169.
27. Bach, B., Mulder, R.T. (2022). Empirical foundation of the ICD-11 Classification of Personality Disorders. In Huprich, S.K. (Ed.), *Personality Disorders and Pathology: Integrating Clinical Assessment and Practice in the DSM-5 and ICD-11 Era*. Washington, DC: American Psychological Association.
28. Somma, A., Gialdi, G., Fossati, A. (2020). Reliability and construct validity of the Personality Inventory for ICD-11 (PiCD) in Italian adult participants. *Psychol Assess*, **32**(1), 29–39.
29. Oltmanns, J.R., Widiger, T.A. (2020). The Five-Factor Personality Inventory for ICD-11: a facet-level assessment of the ICD-11 trait model. *Psychol Assess*, **32**(1), 60–71.
30. Kerber, A., Schultze, M., Müller, S., et al. (2022). Development of a short and ICD-11 compatible measure for DSM-5 maladaptive personality traits using ant colony optimization algorithms. *Assessment*, **29**(3), 467–487.
31. Bach, B., Kerber, A., Aluja, A., et al. (2020). International assessment of DSM-5 and ICD-11 personality disorder traits: toward a common nosology in DSM-5.1. *Psychopathology*, **53**(3-4), 179–188.
32. Skodol, A.E., Clark, L.A., Bender, D.S., et al. (2011). Proposed changes in personality and personality disorder assessment and diagnosis for DSM-5 Part I:

description and rationale. *Personal Disord*, **2**(1), 4–22.

33. Chamberlain, S.R., Stochl, J., Redden, S.A., Grant, J.E. (2018). Latent traits of impulsivity and compulsivity: toward dimensional psychiatry. *Psychol Med*, **48**(5), 810–821.

34. Hopwood, C.J., Kotov, R., Krueger, R.F., et al. (2018). The time has come for dimensional personality disorder diagnosis. *Personal Ment Health*, **12**(1), 82–86.

35. Tyrer, P. (2009). Why borderline personality disorder is neither borderline nor a personality disorder. *Personal Ment Health*, **3**(2), 86–95.

36. Sharp, C. (2016). Current trends in BPD research as indicative of a broader sea-change in psychiatric nosology. *Personal Disord*, **7**(4), 334–343.

37. Mulder, R.T., Horwood, L.J., Tyrer, P. (2020). The borderline pattern descriptor in the International Classification of Diseases, 11th Revision: a redundant addition to classification. *Aust NZ J Psychiatry*, **54**(11), 1095–1100.

38. Herpertz, S.C., Huprich, S.K., Bohus, M., et al. (2017). The challenge of transforming the diagnostic system of personality disorders. *J Pers Disord*, **31**(5), 577–589.

39. Tyrer, P., Mulder, R.T., Kim, Y.R., Crawford, M.J. (2019). The development of the ICD-11 classification of personality disorders: an amalgam of science, pragmatism, and politics. *Annu Rev Clin Psychol*, **15**, 481–502.

40. Chanen, A.M., McCutcheon, L. (2013). Prevention and early intervention for borderline personality disorder: current status and recent evidence. *Br J Psychiatry*, **202** (S54: Youth mental health: appropriate service response to emerging evidence), S24–S29.

41. Blum, N., St John, D., Pfohl, B., et al. (2008). Systems Training for Emotional Predictability and Problem Solving (STEPPS) for outpatients with borderline personality disorder: a randomized controlled trial and 1-year follow-up. *Am J Psychiatry*, **165**(4), 468–478.

42. Zanarini, M.C., Frankenburg, F.R., Reich, D.B., Fitzmaurice, G. (2012). Attainment and stability of sustained symptomatic remission and recovery among patients with borderline personality disorder and axis II comparison subjects: a 16-year prospective follow-up study. *Am J Psychiatry*, **169**(5), 476–483.

43. Lieb, K., Völlm, B., Rücker, G., Timmer, A., Stoffers, J.M. (2010). Pharmacotherapy for borderline personality disorder: Cochrane systematic review of randomised trials. *Br J Psychiatry*, **196**(1), 4–12.

44. Duggan, C., Huband, N., Smailagic, N., Ferriter, M., Adams, C. (2008). The use of pharmacological treatments for people with personality disorder: a systematic review of randomized controlled trials. *Personal Ment Health*, **2**(3), 119–170.

45. Mulder, R.T., Bach, B. (2022). Assessment and treatment of PDs within the ICD-11 Framework. In Huprich, S.K. (Ed.), *Personality Disorders and Pathology: Integrating Clinical Assessment and Practice in the DSM-5 and ICD-11 Era*. Washington, DC: American Psychological Association.

46. Tyrer, P., Mulder, R.T. (2018). Dissecting the elements of borderline personality disorder. *Personal Ment Health*, **12**(2), 91–92.

47. Tyrer, P., Mulder, R. (2022). *Personality Disorder: From Evidence to Understanding*. Cambridge: Cambridge University Press.

48. Nutt, D., Glue, P. (1989). Monoamine oxidase inhibitors: rehabilitation from recent research? *Br J Psychiatry*, **154**, 287–291.

49. Grant, J.E., Baldwin, D.S., Chamberlain, S.R. (2021). Time to reconsider monoamine oxidase inhibitors for obsessive compulsive disorder? A case series using phenelzine. *J Clin Psychopharmacol*, **41**, 461–464.

Chapter 10

Disorders of Intellectual Development

Sally-Ann Cooper & Cary S. Kogan

Introduction

The ICD-11 for mortality and morbidity statistics (ICD-11)[1] classifies disorders of intellectual development within the group of neurodevelopmental disorders. The term 'disorders of intellectual development' reflects a name change from 'mental retardation', which was used in the ICD-10 classification of mental and behavioural disorders (ICD-10).[2] This is an important advance, as language evolves, and the former term has become stigmatized. Disorders of intellectual development have been included in ICD-11, as well as their consequences being included in the World Health Organization's (WHO) *International Classification of Functioning, Disability, and Health* (ICF).[3] This is important, as global statistical returns to the WHO are made using ICD, and so this reinforces the global focus on the importance of addressing the needs of people with disorders of intellectual development. The term is helpful to enable each individual's needs to be assessed and described, so that appropriate access to services can be put in place and appropriate provision of service can be identified at a population level.

Semantics continually change and progress, and individuals and their families and services have their own preferences to describe their disorders and needs. This can lead to considerable confusion in cross-communication locally and internationally. As clinicians and scientists, we advocate that in appropriate settings, language should be used that has clear, operationalized definitions in the classificatory systems, which in the case of ICD-11 is disorders of intellectual development.

Essential Features

The essential features of disorders of intellectual development can be summarized as the following:

- Significant limitations in intellectual functioning across a range of domains, for example perceptual reasoning, working memory, processing speed, and verbal comprehension. The extent of the limitations can, and often does, vary across the domains.
- Significant limitations in adaptive behaviour/daily living skills, across conceptual, social, and practical domains.
- Onset during the developmental period (which, if necessary, can be assessed retrospectively).

Further detail on the essential features is provided in ICD-11. Significant limitations are defined as approximately more than two standard deviations lower than the mean, and preferably are assessed using standardized tests of intellectual and adaptive functioning.

When conducting such assessments, it is important to take account of the context around the individual's development and ability to complete testing, including additional disorders and impairments, culture, first language, environment, opportunities, and extent of training. If standardized tests are not available for use within the responsible health care system, then comprehensive clinical assessment is important. The new ICD-11 tables on intellectual functioning and adaptive behaviour functioning at the different levels of mild, moderate, severe, and profound disorders of intellectual development at different developmental ages (early childhood, childhood and adolescence, and adulthood) should be a helpful guide. It is also essential to reflect that a person's environment may impact on the extent to which their disorder of intellectual development impairs their functioning, for example living and working in a highly technical society or in a low-tech rural society, and the extent of support and training they receive. Additionally, these factors all contribute such that the outcomes of an assessment at one point of time may not necessarily reflect outcomes at a future point of time.

Levels of Intellectual Development Disorder

6A00. Disorders of intellectual development are specified as:
- 6A00.0 Mild disorder of intellectual development; approximately 2–3 standard deviations below mean intellectual functioning, and adaptive behaviour functioning
- 6A00.1 Moderate disorder of intellectual development; approximately 3–4 standard deviations below mean intellectual functioning, and adaptive behaviour functioning
- 6A00.2 Severe disorder of intellectual development; approximately 4+ standard deviations below mean intellectual functioning, and adaptive behaviour functioning
- 6A00.3 Profound disorder of intellectual development; approximately 4+ standard deviations below mean intellectual functioning, and adaptive behaviour functioning
- 6A00.4 Disorder of intellectual development, provisional; this is a provisional diagnosis used under the age of 4, or older if it a valid assessment cannot be undertaken due to other disorders or impairments
- 6A00.Z Disorders of intellectual development, unspecified

In view of intellectual test limitations, severe and profound disorders of intellectual functioning should be delineated on the basis of adaptive behaviour functioning.

The four behavioural indicators tables give examples at the different levels of disorder of intellectual development, and age to aid assessments in the absence of standardized tests, for example in low- and middle-income countries. They have been tested as follows. Adaptive behaviour functioning was studied using a dataset of 658 Italians with disorders of intellectual development: 60 aged up to 6 years, 171 aged 6–18 years, and 427 aged 18+ years. Level of intellectual development was known for 466 of the individuals; 20.1% had a mild, 21.0% had a moderate, 24.5% had a severe, and 5.3% had a profound disorder of intellectual development. Cluster analysis was undertaken on their Vineland II Scale (Italian adaptation)[4] scores across three domains (communication skills, social skills, and daily living skills), and the sample was then split, analyses repeated, and cross-validation undertaken using the kappa coefficient. The agreement was very good or excellent for the 6- to 18-year-olds (ranging from 0.77 to 0.94 across domains) and the 18+-year-olds (ranging from 0.86 to 0.93), and moderate to very good in the 0- to 5-year-olds (0.58–0.63).[5] A subsequent international field trial has shown inter-rater reliability to be excellent (ranging from 0.91 to 0.97) and concurrent validity with standardized measures (i.e., Leiter-3 and Vineland Adaptive Behavior Scales-II) to be good to excellent (Inter Class Correlations: 0.66–0.82).[6]

The coding rule is that clinicians should code the disorder at the most specific level, so technically the general category of 6A00 disorders of intellectual development should not be used, as it is the overarching term referring to the family of disorders. The code *6A00.Z disorders of intellectual development, unspecified* can be used, but best practice is to specify the degree of the disorder. An example of a good use of 'unspecified' is when a person coding diagnoses in electronic health systems is unsure about the clinician's intended diagnosis.

There are numerous aetiologies that result in disorders of intellectual development. When a disorder of intellectual development is diagnosed, it is important to investigate additionally its aetiology, as different aetiologies require differing care both in the short and long term. Both the disorder of intellectual development and its aetiology can and should be classified using ICD-11. Given that multi-morbidity is typical in people with disorders of intellectual development, it is also important to undertake thorough assessment for other physical and mental disorders and additionally classify these, so that these can be optimally treated and supported.

Co-morbidities

Co-morbidities are briefly considered in ICD-11. These vary considerably between people (as do their personalities), though typically people with disorders of intellectual development have multi-morbidity and complex morbidity.[7,8] This adds complexity to diagnostic assessments and interventions for co-morbidities. In its discussion on co-morbidities, ICD-11 focuses mainly on mental disorders and problem behaviours. It highlights that presentations differ depending on degree of intellectual development, age, and other personal factors, and some disorders occur more commonly than in other people, for example, autism spectrum disorder, schizophrenia, bipolar disorder, and dementia. Problem behaviours are also common, while other conditions such as depression and anxiety are also commonly experienced (as they are in other people).

There are many aetiologies of disorders of intellectual development, and some of these have associated behavioural (and physical) phenotypes (types of behaviours and disorders that are more common in the population with a particular underlying aetiology than in other populations), though not everyone with a particular type of aetiology will have all of the disorders associated with the phenotype. Examples are affective psychosis (not an ICD-11 term), self-injurious behaviour, and failure of satiety leading to obesity (and its sequelae such as diabetes) in people with Prader–Willi syndrome; dementia, thyroid dysfunction, and congenital heart disorders in people with Down syndrome; and epilepsies and hypertension (and its sequelae) in people with tuberous sclerosis.

In addition to co-morbidity with mental, behavioural, and other neurodevelopmental disorders, it is also important to be aware of and consider the physical disorders and sensory impairments that are typically present in people with disorders of intellectual development; multi-morbidity is normal in this population. The practitioners who are providing assessments, interventions, and support for this population should also consider each individual's wider needs, including their physical health, and do so within the context of their family and other supports, their vulnerabilities, and their strengths. Multi-morbidity renders assessments and treatments more complex, particularly within the context of limitations in two-way reciprocal communication and additional visual and hearing impairments, and so need to be individualized according to needs. Further complexity results from the drug–drug, drug–disease, and disease–disease adverse interactions that can occur due to multi-morbidity, and from prescribing for multiple individual disorders. This may be especially challenging for practitioners with limited experience/training devoted to these issues. Even in countries with highly resourced health and care systems, this can result in poorer care than for other people,[9,10] and contribute to the premature mortality experienced by the population with disorders of intellectual development through over-representation of avoidable deaths.[11] The pattern of common physical disorders in the population with disorders of intellectual development differs from that seen in the general population, and includes conditions that are painful, disabling, and/or life threatening. Examples include epilepsies, aspiration and respiratory infections, gastrointestinal reflux disorder, constipation, obesity (and its sequalae), and dental disorders, all of which occur both more commonly and with greater severity/complexity than in the general population. When using the ICD-11, coding all co-morbidities is usually clinically relevant, for example in communications between specialist services and primary care.

Diagnostic Boundaries from Normality and Other Disorders

Differential diagnosis of disorders of intellectual development includes differentiating from other neurodevelopmental disorders, other mental disorders and their psychotropic treatments, and physical disorders, and, especially in young children, sensory impairments such as being deaf. It should be noted that these disorders can occur co-morbidly, as well as needing to be considered as part of a differential diagnosis. These can all impact on scores attained on an intelligence quotient test. Scores can also be impacted by, for example, the testing environment, testing persons not in their first language/culture, temporary ill health, and poor concentration for other reasons; such scores alone therefore should not be a sole means of diagnosis, and would not meet the ICD-11 essential features. Intelligence quotient test results can also have poor validity when children have experienced extreme poverty of environment. This can require considerable clinical interpretation. Changes may also occur over time, as children and young people gradually learn and acquire skills, and their support requirements can improve over time.

The main examples to consider in differential diagnosis include:
- Autism spectrum disorders. These conditions often co-occur, while the core features of each disorder differ. Individuals with autism spectrum disorders have impairments in reciprocal social interaction and social communication (among other challenges), but, unless they additionally have a disorder of intellectual development, they do not have the same breadth of limitations across intellectual and adaptive functioning domains. The codes for ICD-11 autism spectrum disorder deliberately incorporate specifiers for presence or absence of disorders of intellectual development (in addition to the separate codes for disorders of intellectual development) when there is assumed shared aetiology. While this approach is not adopted across the other neurodevelopmental disorders, for example disorder of intellectual development and epilepsies, it may aid clinical practice. The codes which include disorder of intellectual development are:
    ○ 6A02.1 Autism spectrum disorder, with disorder of intellectual development, with mild or no impairment of functional language
    ○ 6A02.3 Autism spectrum disorder, with disorder of intellectual development, with impaired functional language

- 6A02.5 Autism spectrum disorder, with disorder of intellectual development, with complete, or almost complete, absence of functional language
- Developmental speech and language disorders. The distinction to be made here is between disorders of reception, expression, articulation, and/or fluency, rather than the more global breadth of limitations across intellectual and adaptive functioning domains that are essential for disorders of intellectual development.
- Developmental learning disorders. The distinction here is between significant limitations in learning specific academic skills of reading, writing, and/or arithmetic despite academic instruction, rather than the more global breadth of limitations across intellectual and adaptive functioning domains that are essential for disorders of intellectual development.
- Other mental, behavioural, or neurodevelopmental disorders, physical disorders including sensory impairments, and medication with psychotropic drugs. In particular, differentiating between impairments due to long-standing schizophrenia and disorders of intellectual development in the absence of collateral or other developmental history can be challenging if required in adulthood, and screening for hearing impairment in young children with developmental delay is essential.

Changes from ICD-10

The main changes from ICD-10 are:
- The name change from mental retardation to disorders of intellectual development.
- Coding hierarchy changes, including an overarching term of 'disorders of intellectual development', followed by specifiers to describe the disorder as 'mild disorder of intellectual development', 'moderate disorder of intellectual development', 'severe disorder of intellectual development', 'profound disorder of intellectual development', 'disorder of intellectual development, provisional', or 'disorder of intellectual development, unspecified'. In ICD-10, the hierarchy is 'mild mental retardation', 'moderate mental retardation', 'severe mental retardation', 'profound mental retardation', 'unspecified mental retardation', and 'other mental retardation', followed by specifiers for impairment of behaviour. The over-arching term 'disorders of intellectual development' should not be used for coding. It is in the plural as it refers to the five specified and one unspecified disorders. The specified disorders, such as mild disorder of intellectual development, are in the singular, and these cover a range of developmental domains as is highlighted in the tables.
- The removal of the optional specifier to mental retardation of 'no, or minimal, impairment in behaviour', 'significant impairment of behaviour requiring attention or treatment', 'other impairments of behaviour', or 'without mention of impairment of behaviour'. There is no equivalent in ICD-11.
- The categories of mild, moderate, severe, or profound disorder of intellectual development no longer provide intelligence quotient ranges, and instead allow for clinical judgement by referring to approximate numbers of standard deviations lower than the mean for intelligence and adaptive behaviour on standard tests or percentile of the population.
- The introduction of tables giving examples of behavioural indicators of intellectual functioning for each of mild, moderate, severe, and profound disorder of intellectual

development for children, children and adolescents, and adults; and tables on conceptual, social, and practical adaptive behaviour indicators at mild, moderate, severe, and profound disorders of intellectual development for children up to age 6, children and adolescents aged 6–18, and adults aged over 18 years. A thorough evidence-based process was used to develop these indicators. In ICD-10, the examples given are discussive rather than tabulated.
- More detailed bullet-pointed content on co-morbidities, differential diagnosis, course, and consideration of cultural and other contextual, appropriateness of tests and norms, as opposed to the discussive format in ICD-10.
- Specification in the over-arching paragraph on 'neurodevelopmental disorders' that the developmental period is typically up to age 18; this is not specified in the section on 'disorders of intellectual development', though prior to ICD-11 this was typically taken to refer to up to the age of 16 years.

Comparison with DSM-5

The developers of ICD-11 worked with those of the *Diagnostic and Statistical Manual of Mental Disorders*, 5th edition (DSM-5)[12] to improve harmonization between the two classification systems, particularly of the metastructure. They reported good agreement on the metastructure for neurodevelopmental disorders, and only minor differences with regard to disorders of intellectual development.[13] Differences are:
- The name used for the disorder. DSM-5 refers to 'intellectual disabilities' in the over-arching title, then 'intellectual disability (intellectual developmental disorder)' in the further detail. This reflects the disparity in publication date between the two manuals, and the spirit of harmonization, as intellectual developmental disorders was the earlier working title used by the ICD-11 working group at the time of publication of DSM-5.[14]
- The hierarchy also differs, although the concepts are similar, with ICD-11 coding disorders of intellectual development using the specifiers of 'mild', 'moderate', 'severe', 'profound', and 'provisional'. DSM-5 is more similar to ICD-10, coding 'mild', 'moderate', 'severe', and 'profound' intellectual disability, 'global developmental delay', and 'unspecified intellectual disability (intellectual developmental disorder)', rather than these being specifiers. The diagnosis of global developmental delay is similar to that in ICD-11 of 'disorder of intellectual development, provisional', though DSM-5 reserves the diagnosis for children under the age of 5, while ICD-11 refers to infants or children under the age of 4, or older if valid assessments cannot be conducted due to other disorders or impairments. DSM-5 unspecified intellectual disability refers to individuals over the age of 5 in whom assessment of degree of intellectual disability is not possible locally due to associated sensory or physical impairments, while ICD-11 does not describe when it should be used, on the assumption that the degree of the disorder will be specified.
- The table on severity levels for 'intellectual disability (intellectual developmental disorder)' in DSM-5 includes the same domains of conceptual, social, and practical skills used in the ICD-11 tables on adaptive functioning. It is more concise and less standardized than the tables in ICD-11, and not field-tested. ICD-11 and DSM-5 provide different examples in their tables to convey similar meaning.

- DSM-5 does not provide a table on intellectual functioning, so while its diagnostic criteria include 'deficits' in both intellectual and adaptive functioning, severity is based just on adaptive functioning.
- ICD-11 provides more information on co-morbidities, differential diagnosis, course, and consideration of cultural and other contextual appropriateness of tests and norms than does DSM-5, where these considerations are more concisely addressed. DSM-5 considers 'associated features', such as social judgement, assessment of risk, self-management of behaviour, emotions, or interpersonal relationships, motivation, gullibility, and exploitation, while the 'additional features' section in ICD-11 focuses more on co-morbidities, though it also touches on gullibility, exploitation, and life events.

Advantages of ICD-11

The advantages of ICD-11 over ICD-10 and from its differences with DSM-5 will become more apparent once ICD-11 enters general usage. At this stage, we suggest that there are two likely advantages:

- The name change from 'mental retardation' to 'disorders of intellectual development'. Language continually evolves, and the term 'mental retardation', which was introduced several decades ago, is now considered stigmatizing, so is very unhelpful to individuals and their families. Internationally, the term 'intellectual disabilities' is currently in common usage academically and professionally, and is the DSM-5 term (though used in the singular form of 'intellectual disability'). The family of classification systems used by the World Health Organization precluded this term as the classification of disability is included as part of a separate classification, the International Classification of Functioning, Disability and Health (ICF). The difference is explained by the need in ICD-11 to separate the nature of disorders from their functional consequences. The careful considerations relating to this point are likely to benefit people with disorders of intellectual disabilities and their families in future, as it means their needs remain included in the ICD-11 classification which is used for statistical returns by almost all nations globally. At a population level these needs will be reported so cannot be ignored.
- While there are several existing scales that measure intellectual functioning and adaptive functioning, training in their use and highly trained professionals to administer them are not always universally accessible. Barriers may also include lack of translation to local languages and lack of standardization and norms for some populations. The tables on behavioural indicators of intellectual and adaptive functioning provided in ICD-11 and in the associated academic publication[5] are therefore a considerable advantage in terms of access to this information to aid diagnosis.

There are two points requiring further consideration, which could perhaps be addressed in future through the ICD-11 iteration processes. These are:

- Problem behaviours. The problem behaviours optional specifiers to mental retardation in ICD-10 of 'no, or minimal, impairment in behaviour', 'significant impairment of behaviour requiring attention or treatment', 'other impairments of behaviour', or 'without mention of impairment of behaviour' no longer exist in ICD-11, and so it will not be possible for the WHO to know their prevalence. The focus behind the revision of

ICD (see Chapter 1) was clinical utility, so once ICD-11 is in general usage, if the specification of problem behaviours emerges as something that would be regarded as clinically useful, it will then be added in a subsequent revision.
- The further confusion of terminology (from the perspective of people with disorders of intellectual development, their families, practitioners, and academics) regarding the introduction of the term 'developmental learning disorders' (referred to as 'specific learning disorder' in DSM-5) and previously termed as 'specific developmental disabilities' in ICD-10 (and 'learning disorders' in DSM-IV[15]). Additionally, within the ICD-11 subcategories of these disorders, the terms 'learning difficulties' and 'learning impairments' are used for developmental learning disorders. Unfortunately, these terms are currently used simultaneously for what ICD-11 classifies as 'disorders of intellectual development' in education, health and social care, national policy, and law in some countries (especially in the UK, where services have not changed their language descriptions). This extends the likelihood of confusion/error in classification and in everyday cross-communication, which ideally classification should avoid, as it is aimed at producing statistics to benefit people needing services and support.

Problem Behaviours

We use the term 'problem behaviour' in this chapter to be synonymous with other terms used internationally such as challenging behaviour, behaviour which challenges, and behaviour disorders. There are pros and cons for each of these diagnostic terms. Problem behaviours are markedly disruptive, recurrent behaviours which are noticeably out of keeping with the person's social and cultural background, environment, and age, and which interfere with the person's quality of life or health and safety or that of others. They present across a range of personal and social situations, although may be more severe in certain identified settings. Statistical research on psychopathology experienced by people with disorders of intellectual development provides evidence on their worth and validity.[16]

Problem behaviours are important to consider for people with disorders of intellectual development, as they are common, affect families, are very disabling, and require interventions and support from services, incurring both individual and societal costs. They can impact the adult when integrating with, and participating in, the local community and in accessing resources, pose problems maintaining social networks, may exclude the individual from services, cause a breakdown of support packages, and impact self-esteem. They can also have negative consequences for family and paid carers, including injury and carer-strain. They are the most common cause for referral to mental health services for people with disorders of intellectual development (e.g., accounting for about 50 per cent of such referrals in the UK) and for breakdown of residential support packages.

The ICD-10 category of mental retardation included an optional specifier on problem behaviours of 'no, or minimal, impairment in behaviour', 'significant impairment of behaviour requiring attention or treatment', 'other impairments of behaviour', or 'without mention of impairment of behaviour'. WHO also produced a guide to provide additional information on mental retardation, including common types of impaired behaviour.[17] This optional specifier has now been removed in ICD-11.

The ICD-10 specifier lacked any granular detail of the person's problem behaviours, and so was limited. Its removal means that statistical returns and local analyses will not include it. Clinicians will likely either diagnose the person as having a disorder of intellectual development and omit the reason for the consultation, or attempt to capture the reason for consulting health services with another category in ICD-11 including using 'unspecified' categories, none of which really captures the nature of the problem behaviours experienced, given the associated emotional dysregulation and distress incurred by the individual.

Guiding principles in the development of a revised ICD were to address 'clinically recognisable sets of symptoms or behaviours associated in most cases with distress and with interference with personal functions', and to consider 'how a diagnosis and classification manual can assist an increase coverage and enhance mental health care across the world'. These principles could be applied to problem behaviours. Inclusion in ICD-11, for example by a more detailed specifier than that in ICD-10, would have enabled guidance for the development of individual treatments/interventions/support plans; prognostic guidance regarding long-term support needs, aided research on epidemiology, protective and vulnerability factors, experimental studies, and trials; raised visibility in government statistics; and enabled international communication and comparisons. It is a pity that ICD-11 will be deficient in this regard.

Several types of disorder with prominent behaviours are included within ICD-11. In some cases, they may be suitable to use with people with disorders of intellectual development who have problem behaviours. Many (e.g., oppositional defiant disorder, aggressive behaviour, and non-suicidal self-injury) require insight into the person's mental state such as their urges, intentions, deliberate intent, deliberate defiance, and spitefulness, which are often uncertain or not present, particularly in people with more severe disorders of intellectual development, who are most likely to experience problem behaviours. Most also do not capture the individual's type of distress associated with their problem behaviour, which is often pronounced. Within ICD-11, examples include: Mental, behavioural, or neurodevelopmental disorders:

- Neurodevelopmental disorders
  - 6A06.0 Stereotyped movement disorder
    - 6A06.1 Stereotyped movement disorder with self-injury
  - 6E60 Secondary neurodevelopmental syndrome
- Obsessive-compulsive or related disorders
  - 6B24 Hoarding disorder
- Feeding or eating disorders
  - 6B84 Pica
  - 6B85 Rumination–regurgitation disorder
  - 6B8Y Other specified feeding or eating disorders
  - 6B8Z Feeding or eating disorders, unspecified
- Elimination disorders
  - 6C00 Enuresis
  - 6C01 Encopresis
  - 6C0Z Elimination disorders, unspecified

- Impulse control disorders
    - 6C70 Pyromania
    - 6C71 Kleptomania
    - 6C72 Compulsive sexual behaviour disorder
    - 6C73 Intermittent explosive disorder
    - 6B25 Body-focused repetitive behaviour disorders
        - 6B25.0 Trichotillomania
        - 6B25.1 Excoriation disorder
        - 6B25.Y Other specified body-focused repetitive behaviour disorders
        - 6B25.Z Body focused repetitive disorders, unspecified
    - 6C7Y Other specified impulse control disorders
    - 6C7Z Impulse control disorders, unspecified
- Disruptive behaviour or dissocial disorders
    - 6C90 Oppositional defiant disorder
    - 6C90.0 Oppositional defiant disorder, with chronic irritability-anger
        - 6C90.00 with limited prosocial emotions
        - 6C90.01 with typical prosocial emotions
        - 6C90.0Z unspecified
    - 6C90.1 Oppositional defiant disorder, without chronic irritability-anger
        - 6C90.10 with limited prosocial emotions
        - 6C90.11 with typical prosocial emotions
        - 6C90.1Z unspecified
    - 6C90.Z Oppositional defiant disorder, unspecified
    - 6C91 Conduct-dissocial disorder
        - 6C91.0 Conduct-dissocial disorder, childhood onset
        - 6C91.1 Conduct-dissocial disorder, adolescent onset
        - 6C91.Z Conduct-dissocial disorder, unspecified
    - 6C9Y Other specified disruptive behaviour or dissocial disorder
    - 6C9Z Disruptive behaviour or dissocial disorders, unspecified,
- Paraphilic disorders
    - 6D30 Exhibitionistic disorder
    - 6D31 Voyeuristic disorder
    - 6D32 Pedophilic disorder
    - 6D34 Frotteuristic disorder
    - 6D3Z Paraphilic disorders, unspecified

Diseases of the digestive system:

- Functional gastrointestinal disorders
    - DD90 Functional oesophageal or gastroduodenal disorders

- DD90.6 Adult rumination syndrom
- DD90.Y Other specified functional oesophageal or gastroduodenal disorders,
- DD90.Z Functional oesophageal or gastroduodenal disorders, unspecified

Symptoms, signs or clinical findings, not elsewhere classified:

- MB23 Symptoms or signs involving appearance or behaviour
  - MB23.0 Aggressive behaviour
  - MB23.E Non-suicidal self-injury

ICD-11 also includes the 'catch-all' categories of:

- 6E8Y Other specified mental, behavioural or neurodevelopmental disorders
- 6E8Z Mental, behavioural or neurodevelopmental disorders, unspecified

As the ICD-11 is gradually introduced into clinical usage, the utility or otherwise of these above categories for people with disorders of intellectual developmental will become more apparent.

Discussion

Important progress has been made in changing ICD-11 from ICD-10, in particular the name change from one that had become stigmatizing and unacceptable to people with the disorder and their families, and so had fallen into disuse. The tables on both intellectual and adaptive behaviour functioning should be a useful aid to diagnosis when standardized test materials are not available. Once ICD-11 is introduced into common practice, further advantages will become clearer over time.

Two issues remain pertinent for further consideration: problem behaviours and the diagnosis of other mental, behavioural, and neurodevelopmental disorders experienced by people with disorders of intellectual development.

Problem behaviours are common, distressing, and burdensome to the individual and their families, and are the main reason for presentation of people with disorders of intellectual development to mental health services. Addition of specifiers that can be used to code problem behaviours alongside a diagnosis of disorder of intellectual development provides a possible direction for how ICD-11 could iterate to address their current omission.

With respect to other mental, behavioural, or neurodevelopmental disorders experienced by people with disorders of intellectual development, diagnosis is more complex than for most (but not all) other people. This is due to many factors, including disabilities, impairments, communication, and the cognitive level needed to understand and describe concepts, and a greater reliance on collateral reporting (often from multiple carers). For several reasons, standard classificatory systems perform less well when used with people with disorders of intellectual development, for example the range of psychopathology within disorders differs compared with the general population (dementia is an example), and general population criteria tend to rely on verbal items and intellectually complex concepts that are lacking when intellectual function is impaired. Disorders often have detailed subcategorization, and this increases the potential for diagnostic error when extrapolating their use to people with disorders of intellectual development; approaches to classification can be particularly complicated when coding for people who have syndromes with associated behavioural phenotypes. Often this results in use of the residual 'unspecified' categories.

It will become clearer over time as ICD-11 enters into general usage if these factors impact on the utility of ICD-11 for this population. In view of these issues, the UK Royal College of Psychiatrists previously produced a manual to be used alongside ICD-10 to assist clinicians in using ICD-10 criteria with people with disorders of intellectual development: the *DC-LD: Diagnostic Criteria for Psychiatric Disorders for Use with Adults with Learning Disabilities/Mental Retardation.*[18] DC-LD also included descriptions of classifications of problem behaviours, and in additional work developed a rating scale for the measurement of problem behaviours suitable for use in research.[19] Work in the USA has also produced further detail on the use of DSM-5 for people with disorders of intellectual development.[20] Once the details of ICD-11 are more widely available, a similar complementary manual could be produced for use with people with disorders of intellectual development, if needed.

In summary, ICD-11 provides classificatory advantages over ICD-10 for people with disorders of intellectual development, while further iteration, particularly regarding problem behaviours, might bring more individual and societal benefits.

References

1. World Health Organization. (1992). *The ICD-10 Classification of Mental and Behavioural Disorders. Clinical Descriptions and Diagnostic Guidelines*. Geneva: World Health Organization.

2. World Health Organization. (2018). *ICD-11*. [Available from: https://icd.who.int/.]

3. World Health Organization. (2001). *International Classification of Functioning, Disability, and Health*. Geneva: World Health Organization.

4. Balboni, G., Belacchi, C., Bonichini, S., et al. (2016). *Vineland-II. Vineland Adaptive Behaviour Scales Second Edition. Survey Interview Form. Standardizzazione Italiana*. Florence: Giunti OS.

5. Tasse, M.J., Balboni, G.P. (2019). Developing behavioural indicators for intellectual functioning and adaptive behaviour for ICD-11 disorders of intellectual development. *J Intellect Disabil Res*, **63**, 386–407.

6. Lemay, K.R., Kogan, C.S., Rebello, T.J., et al. (2022). An international field study of the ICD-11 behavioural indicators for disorders of intellectual development. *J Intellect Disabil Res*, **66**(4), 376–391.

7. Cooper, S-A., McLean, G., Guthrie, B., et al. (2015). Multiple physical and mental health comorbidity in adults with intellectual disabilities: population-based cross-sectional analysis. *BMC Fam Pract*, **16**, 110.

8. Kinnear, D., Morrison, J., Allan, L., et al. (2018). The prevalence of multi-morbidity in a cohort of adults with intellectual disabilities, with and without Down syndrome. *BMJ Open*, **8**, e018292,.

9. Hanlon, P., Wood, K., Cooper, S-A., et al. (2018). Long-term condition management in adults with intellectual disability in primary care: a systematic review. *BJGP Open*, **2**(1), bjgpopen18X101445.

10. Hughes-McCormack, L., Greenlaw, N., McSkimming, P., et al. (2021). Trends over time in the management of long-term conditions in primary health care for adults with intellectual disabilities, and the health care inequality gap with the general population. *J Appl Res Intellect Disabil*, **34**, 634–637.

11. Heslop, P., Blair, P.S., Fleming, P., et al. (2014). The confidential inquiry into premature deaths of people with intellectual disabilities in the UK: a population based study. *Lancet*, **383**, 889–895.

12. American Psychiatric Association. (2013). *Diagnostic and Statistical Manual of Mental Disorders*, 5th ed. Arlington, VA: American Psychiatric Association.

13. First, M.B., Gaebel, W., Maj, M., et al. (2021). An organization- and category-level comparison of diagnostic requirements for mental disorders in ICD-11 and DSM-5. *World Psychiatry*, **20**, 34–51.

14. Salvador-Carulla, L., Reed, G.M., Vaez-Azizi, L.M., et al. (2011). Intellectual developmental disorders: towards a new name, definition and framework for 'mental retardation/intellectual disability' in ICD-11. *World Psychiatry*, **10**, 175–80.
15. American Psychiatric Association. *Diagnostic and Statistical Manual of Mental Disorders*, 4th ed. Washington, DC: American Psychiatric Association, 1994.
16. Melville, C., McConnachie, A., Johnson, P., et al. (2016). Problem behaviours and symptom dimensions of psychiatric disorders in adults with intellectual disabilities: an exploratory and confirmatory factor analysis. *Res Developmental Disabil*, **55**, 1–13.
17. World Health Organization. (1996). *ICD-10 Guide for Mental Retardation*. Geneva: World Health Organization.
18. Royal College of Psychiatrists. (2001). *DC-LD: Diagnostic Criteria for Psychiatric Disorders for Use with Adults with Learning Disabilities/Mental Retardation*. London: Gaskell Press.
19. Tyrer, P., Nagar, J., Evans, R., et al. (2016). The problem behaviour checklist: short scale to assess challenging behaviours. *BJPsych Open*, **2**, 45–49.
20. Fletcher, R., Barnhill, J., Cooper, S-A. (Eds.) (2016). *The Diagnostic Manual – Intellectual Disability 2. A Textbook of Diagnosis of Mental Disorders in Persons with Intellectual Disability*. (DM-ID-2 Textbook.) New York: NADD Press.

Chapter 11

Eating Disorders

Ulrike Schmidt

Editor's note

In the presentations that took place at the Royal College Webinar on 25 and 26 May 2021, there was insufficient time to include one on eating disorders. Subsequently, Professor Ulrike Schmidt has contributed the following piece about binge eating disorder (BED), the condition representing the major change in classification in this group of disorders since ICD-10. This should be taken in conjunction with the more positive comments about binge eating disorder in Chapter 2.

Response to Professor Frances

Professor Frances raises several important points. First, he argues that binge eating is a 'ubiquitous symptom among normals'. The same applies to most other psychiatric symptoms (e.g., anxiety, mood, or substance use), that is, they occur along a spectrum, and beyond a certain point distress, disability, and impairment of functioning are seen as so severe as to constitute a disorder. Growing evidence supports the notion that BED is a complex, multifactorial, and disabling disorder, with genetic, biological, environmental, and psychosocial variables contributing to the onset and maintenance of dysregulated eating and other related behaviours.[1] Untreated, BED is typically longstanding, with obesity and associated metabolic sequelae (e.g., type 2 diabetes, hypertension) and common multiple psychiatric co-morbidities. The standardized mortality ratio is estimated to be 1.5–1.8. It is also of note that having minority status and being exposed to deprivation, violence, and trauma are thought to increase the risk of developing BED.[2] This has led some experts to think of BED as also containing elements of social (in)justice.[3]

Second, Professor Frances is concerned that inclusion of BED in both DSM-5 and ICD-11 will lead to 'overdiagnosis' and 'diet pill popping'. In this respect, he points to the approval of lisdexamphetamine (Vyvanse) by the FDA as a treatment for BED in the USA. What is perhaps most revealing about this comment is that it highlights some of the systemic problems in the US health care system, for example the role of insurance companies, direct-to-consumer advertising, and a lack of socialized medicine. While these systemic problems are real and need to be addressed, it is also important to recognize that international guidance to date unanimously recommends psychological interventions as first-line treatments for BED.[4]

Finally, eating disorders in general, but specifically those associated with binge eating and obesity, are highly stigmatized in that they are seen as trivial and self-inflicted, more so, for example, than mood disorders. To a degree, Prof Frances' arguments (e.g., talking about 'pet projects' and equating the serious, long-lasting, and distressing symptoms of BED with the occasional over-indulgence in food seen in most people) could be perceived by some as reflecting these attitudes.

References

1. Giel, K.E., Bulik, C.M., Fernandez-Aranda, F., et al. (2022). Binge eating disorder. *Nat Rev Dis Primers*, **8**(1), 16. https://doi.org/10.1038/s41572-022-00344-y
2. Keski-Rahkonen, A. (2021). Epidemiology of binge eating disorder: prevalence, course, comorbidity, and risk factors. *Curr Opin Psychiatry*, **34**(6), 525–531.
3. Bray, B., Bray, C., Bradley, R., Zwickey, H. (2022). Binge eating disorder is a social justice issue: a cross-sectional mixed-methods study of binge eating disorder experts' opinions. *Int J Environ Res Public Health*, **19**(10), 6243.
4. Hilbert, A., Hoek, H.W., Schmidt, R. (2017). Evidence-based clinical guidelines for eating disorders: international comparison. *Curr Opin Psychiatry*, **30**(6), 423–437

Chapter 12

Mental Health Classifications in Primary Care

Christopher Dowrick

Editor's note
There is currently no equivalent of the Primary Care version of ICD-10 in ICD-11, but it is being prepared. This chapter therefore summarizes other current classifications commonly used in primary care as well as giving a report of progress with the ICD-11 version.

The Need for Mental Health Classification in Primary Care

The World Organization of Family Doctors (WONCA) has proposed a set of core competencies in primary mental health care, explaining what can reasonably be expected of trained and qualified family doctors, working in primary care settings in any part of the world, when caring for people with mental health problems.[1] Competencies in assessment include the ability to diagnose common mental health problems, distinguish common mental disorders from normal responses to adverse and traumatic events, the awareness of severe psychiatric problems, assessment of risk, and understanding the interactions between physical and mental health. Family doctors are expected to manage the care of people with common mental health problems and the physical health of people with severe mental health problems. They are expected to use a range of available options and resources for care of people with mental health problems and tailor them to patients' and carers' needs: specifically, this includes sharing the care of patients with severe or complex mental health problems with specialist mental health services.

To be fit for purpose a classification system for mental health problems in primary care therefore needs to provide three important things,
a) to differentiate between normality and disease,
b) to clarify interactions between mind and body, and
c) to indicate levels of severity and complexity.

There are currently four classification options available for use in primary mental health care: the Systematized Nomenclature of Medicine Clinical Terms (SNOMED CT); the 5th edition of the *Diagnostic and Statistical Manual of Mental Disorders* (DSM-5); the 3rd edition of the *International Classification of Primary Care* (ICPC-3); and the proposed primary care version of the 11th edition of the *International Classification of Diseases* (ICD-11 PHC). This chapter considers the strengths and limitations of each option, with particular focus on ICD-11 PHC, and suggests strategies to improve nosology and enhance integration of primary and specialist mental health care.

SNOMED CT

SNOMED CT is a structured clinical vocabulary, currently embedded in the electronic record systems used by family doctors and other primary care professionals across the UK. It is also licensed, though less regularly used, in other countries including the USA and Canada. It is proposed as the most comprehensive and precise clinical health terminology in the world.[2] It provides multiple codes, roughly four times as many as DSM-5 and three times as many as ICD-11.

With regard to depression, this term and its derivatives generate a total of 712 matches. These are categorized as findings, such as 'depressed mood'; observable entity, such as 'depression level'; situation, such as 'h/o depression'; and disorder, such as 'depressive disorder'. There is also a category for procedures, for example screening, counselling, or medication review. The category 'depressive disorder' has 39 subcategories in total, ranging alphabetically from acute depressive disorder to stuporous depression; it includes bipolar – current episode depression, dysthymia, and 'on examination depressed'. Of these 39 subgroups, 9 are available for use in primary care electronic systems: agitated depression, reactive (situational) depression, recurrent depression, reactive depressive psychosis, chronic depression, endogenous depression, mild depression, major depressive disorder, and postpartum depression.

Anxiety and related terms generate 527 matches, including 'anxiety' as a finding and 'anxiety disorder' as a disorder. Anxiety disorder has 28 subgroups, of which most are available to primary care users. Variations on generalized anxiety disorder include anxiety neurosis, mixed anxiety and depressive disorder, separation anxiety, and anxiety about behaviour or performance. Social phobia and agoraphobia are specified, as are panic attack, panic disorder, phobia or phobic disorder, fear of flying, feeling tense, feeling nervous, and nervous tension. For children in the UK (but not elsewhere in the world), there are discrete categories of acute stress disorder and stranger anxiety.

SNOMED CT is less specific in relation to the interactions between psyche and soma. Medically unexplained symptoms and somatic syndrome are categorized as findings, while bodily distress disorder is categorized as a disorder.

The main advantage of SNOMED CT for daily clinical practice in primary care is its ease of use, especially when embedded in primary care electronic records. However, its main limitation, for current purposes, is that it is not really a diagnostic classification system at all but a set of descriptions. There are considerable uncertainties regarding its ontological commitment, that is to say, what kind of entity is an instance of a given concept.[3] In the electronic record, 'Problem' is the standard header, but there is no indication as to whether this refers to disorder (the closest term to diagnosis) or to observation, situation, findings, or procedure. This offers considerable clinical latitude, as in the examples of depression and anxiety given above, but comes with no expectation of a formal diagnosis. Nor are there any underlying descriptions of relevant symptoms and signs to guide clinicians towards a particular formulation. Clinical terminology, however structured and comprehensive, is not the same as clinical diagnosis.

DSM-5

The DSM-5 is published by the American Psychiatric Association and serves as the principal authority for psychiatric diagnoses in the USA. Considering its overall value to international classifications for mental health is beyond the scope of this chapter, but there are two elements of relevance to primary care.

The first is the well-reported obfuscation of the boundaries between grief and depression, allowing a diagnosis of major depressive disorder to be made just 2 weeks after a bereavement. While this may enable patient access to treatments in the US insurance-based health care system, there are major concerns about turning grief and other life stresses into mental disorders and the consequent medical intrusion into personal emotions. It adds unnecessary medication and costs and distracts attention and resources from those who really need them.[4] It also leads to considerable confusion for primary care diagnosticians.

Second, in relation to interactions between psyche and soma, the DSM-5 classification of somatic symptom disorder places emphasis on cognitive elements. A diagnosis of somatic symptom disorder can be made if a patient presents one or more somatic symptoms, associated with 'excessive thoughts, feelings, or behaviors related to the somatic symptoms or associated health concerns'.[5] Specifically, for a diagnosis of somatic symptom disorder, at least one of three psychological criteria should be present: health anxiety, disproportionate and persistent concerns about the medical seriousness of the symptoms, and excessive time and energy devoted to the symptoms or health concerns. As we shall see, this formulation is different from both ICD-11 and ICD-11 PHC.

ICPC-3

The third edition of the *International Classification for Primary Care*, endorsed by WONCA, is now commanding considerable attention worldwide. It is already the classification system of choice for general practitioners and other primary care practitioners in Belgium, Brazil, Finland, France, and the Netherlands. It is under serious consideration by primary care in Canada, Denmark, Kazakhstan, and Norway, though in Canada there is currently a choice between introducing ICD-11 or ICPC-3. There is interest from primary care organizations in India and Malaysia, although these are not official national organizations. ICPC-3 is also the preferred classification system for the WHO Primary Health Care team in its drive towards universal health care.

The ICPC-3 is based on content of the primary care consultation. It covers reasons for encounter, including symptoms and complaints, episodes of care, functioning, and social problems.

Patients normally start the consultation with a spontaneous statement on why they visit the health professional. This is called the Reason for Encounter (RFE). It precedes the interaction and interpretation by the practitioner or the patient. The RFE is the literal expression of the reasons why a person enters the consultation room, translated into an ICPC code by the GP. It represents the need for care by that person. The RFE can be presented in the form of symptoms and complaints (*abdominal pain, exhaustion*) but also as self-diagnosed diseases (*I've got the flu*), a problem in an activity (*I cannot work*), or requests for a particular intervention.

After history taking and physical examination, the practitioner makes a diagnosis or assessment that indicates the care episode in which the encounter takes place. The diagnosis or assessment is the practitioner's point of view. Coding health problems or episodes of care should be at the highest level of diagnostic refinement for which the user can be confident and which meets the inclusion criteria for that category. The episode title can be a symptom, a disease or problem, a problem in activity or participation, or a non-disease-related care episode such as visits related to need for immunization, to special screening examination, and to public health promotion. The episode title can never be a process or intervention.

The definition of an episode of care is a health problem or disease dating from its first presentation to a health care provider to the completion of the last encounter for that same health problem.[6]

Functioning is assessed in ICPC-3 using a selected subset of items from the WHO International Classification of Functioning, Disability and Health (ICF), including WHO-DAS 2.0.[7] Social problems are defined as issues within the personal environment or society that make it difficult for people to achieve their full potential. Poverty, unemployment, unequal opportunity, racism, and malnutrition are examples of social problems, as are substandard housing, employment discrimination, and child abuse and neglect. This allows reference to terms such as 'vulnerability' and 'syndemic', referring to biological and social interactions affecting prognosis, treatment, and health policy, of particular relevance to the escalation of mental disorders during a period of global disruption.[8]

Looking specifically at common mental health problems, ICPC-3 has RFE codes for psychological symptoms or complaints, such as feeling anxious, nervous, or tense or feeling sad. Episode of care codes for psychological diagnoses made by the clinician include anxiety disorder or anxiety state, bodily distress or somatization disorder, depressive disorder, and mixed depressive and anxiety disorder. The ICPC-3 also includes medically unexplained symptoms (MUS) as a code for a long-lasting symptom diagnosis.

ICD-11 PHC

The primary care version of ICD-11 remains a work in progress. A WHO advisory group involving clinical academics from psychiatry and primary care has undertaken field trials in four middle-income and one high-income country. They considered 28 disorders covering childhood disorders, psychotic and dysphoric disorders, bodily distress and body function, substance use, personality disorders, and acquired neurocognitive disorders.

In many cases, ICD-11 PHC proposes a simplified version of ICD-11 classifications suitable for primary care settings.

Eating Disorder

One example is eating disorder, defined as a spectrum disorder, with cardinal features of fear of being fat or gaining weight, and extensive efforts to control or reduce weight such as strict dieting, vomiting, use of purgatives, or excessive exercise.

Three subcategories are recognized as in the standard ICD-11 system: binge eating disorder, bulimia nervosa, and anorexia nervosa. Patients may be diagnosed with a *binge eating disorder* when there are recurrent episodes of binge eating at least once a week for 3 months; the disorder may lead to increases in body weight; binge eating is not associated with the recurrent use of inappropriate compensatory behaviour (e.g., purging or induced vomiting); and does not occur exclusively during the course of bulimia nervosa or anorexia nervosa.

Patients with *bulimia nervosa* typically show normal or rapidly fluctuating body weight; binge eating, that is, eating an amount of food that is definitely larger than most people would eat in a similar period of time under similar circumstances; and purging, attempts to eliminate food by self-induced vomiting or misuse of laxatives, diuretics, or other medications.

Patients with *anorexia nervosa* typically have a body mass index (BMI) of less than 17.5 and/or rapid weight loss of more than 0.5 kg per week and an altered perception of body image. Women with anorexia may have amenorrhoea for 3 months or longer (unless they are taking an oral contraceptive). A proportion of patients will also binge and purge.

Comparing ICDC-11 PHC with other classifications of eating disorders highlights both concordance and differences. In addition to these three categories, ICD-11 includes avoidant-restrictive food intake disorder, pica (the compulsive consumption of non-food items), rumination–regurgitation disorder, as well as other specified or unspecified feeding or eating disorders. The ICPC-3 has the same three categories as ICD-11 PHC but also includes pica. SNOMED CT has a total of 19 subcategories of eating disorder, listed alphabetically from anorexia to weight fixation, and includes orthorexia, defined as an unhealthy obsession with healthy eating.

There are also classifications proposed for ICD-11 PHC which differ from those in ICD-11. The two most important are anxious depression and bodily stress syndrome.

Anxious Depression

The ICD-11 PHC proposes a diagnosis of anxious depression if both anxiety and depressive symptoms are present at case level for at least 2 weeks. This differs from ICD-11's mixed depressive and anxiety disorder, where neither set of symptoms, considered separately, is sufficiently severe, numerous, or persistent to justify a diagnosis of another depressive disorder or an anxiety or fear-related disorder. So, whereas ICD-11 would confer separate diagnoses related to anxiety or depression, ICD-11 PHC proposed a single compound diagnosis.

The rationale for the proposed diagnosis of anxious depression is related to its clinical significance and emerges from research conducted during the field trials. In a study conducted in primary care centres in Brazil, China, Mexico, Pakistan, and Spain, practitioners referred patients based on either perceived psychological distress or distressing somatic symptoms to a research assistant who administered a computer-guided diagnostic interview. Complete data were obtained for 2,279 participants. Anxious depression was the most common diagnosis (48%), compared with generalized anxiety disorder (42%) and mixed anxiety and depressive disorder (45%). One-third of those diagnosed with anxious depression had anxiety lasting less than 3 months, but these participants reported as much disability and suicidal ideation as those with longer duration of symptoms.[9]

In separate research, a 30-year follow-up study in Nottingham, UK, found that cothymia (both anxiety and depression diagnoses) had significantly worse prognosis than either panic disorder or generalized anxiety disorder.[10]

There is evidence from surveys conducted during the ICD-11 PHC field trials of support from primary care practitioners for the diagnosis of anxious depression.[11] However, there is concern that the 2-week criterion for caseness runs the same risk as the DSM-5 criterion for major depressive disorder in blurring the boundary between psychiatric disorder and normal reaction to adverse life events. There is also potential for confusion among primary care practitioners, simply because it is different from ICD-11. And the presence of differing criteria may impede plans for effective integration between primary and mental health services.

Bodily Stress Syndrome

The ICD-11 PHC classification of bodily stress syndrome (BSS) specifies the presence of at least three symptoms not explained by known medical pathology and associated with distress or impairment. It also eliminates the requirement that the primary care practitioner makes a judgement about whether the attention devoted to the symptoms is 'excessive'.

Within ICD-11 PHC, BSS is differentiated from *health anxiety*, with the latter characterized by either or both persistent, intrusive ideas or fears of having an illness that cannot be stopped, or only stopped with great difficulty; or intense preoccupation with minor bodily sensations or problems that are misinterpreted as signs of serious disease.

This represents a change from the previous primary care version of ICD-10, where the diagnosis of *medically unexplained somatic complaints* involved negative physical investigations and frequent visits to the practitioner despite these negative findings.

Bodily stress syndrome also differs from the new ICD-11 diagnosis of *bodily distress disorder* (BDD), which relates to bodily symptoms that are distressing and involve excessive attention and perhaps repeated contact with health care. With BDD, if a medical condition is present, the attention is excessive in relation to its nature and progression. Bodily symptoms and associated distress are persistent and associated with significant impairment. Although BDD will typically involve multiple bodily symptoms that may vary over time, there may be a single symptom – usually pain or fatigue – that is associated with the other features of the disorder. The argument in favour of the multi-symptom BSS diagnosis is that this is needed in primary care because single, unexplained somatic symptoms are so common.

The rationale for the proposed ICD-11 PHC diagnosis of BSS is again based on evidence from field trials conducted in primary care. Unlike DSM-5, where emphasis is on cognitive elements, the focus here is on the substantial overlap between somatic and psychological symptoms.

A study involving 587 patients diagnosed by primary care practitioners with either BSS or health anxiety identified a mean of 11 symptoms per patient: 70% had both BSS and health anxiety, 79% had co-occurring diagnoses of anxiety, depression, or both, and 56% had a diagnosis of anxious depression. Levels of disability were high, with a mean WHO-DAS score of 13.12. In a subsequent statistical analysis of 797 patients with somatic complaints and depressive and anxious symptoms, two bi-factor models fitted the data. The first model had all symptoms loaded on a general factor, along with one of three specific depression, anxiety, and somatic factors. The second had a general factor and two specific anxious depression and somatic factors.[13]

In an earlier US-based study, reflecting on the utility or otherwise of DSM classifications of mental disorder in primary settings, 60 family health centre patients free of mental disorders were recruited. They completed monthly quantitative interviews, using multiple rating instruments, concerning the levels of psychiatric symptoms, presence of distress and/or a mental disorder, functional status, support, and stressors. The study found that psychological symptoms and diagnostic disorders varied considerably over time. Distress and subthreshold disorders were often seen in primary care patients, while the crossing of a diagnostic threshold corresponded to extreme levels of psychological symptoms and may therefore represent symptom severity. Psychological symptoms were often linked to physical illness, and the context in which symptoms and disorders develop often produced complex dynamic patterns.[14]

These studies conclude that mood and anxiety disorders are likely in the presence of multiple somatic symptoms, and suggest that depressive, anxious, and somatic symptoms are best understood as different presentations of a common latent phenomenon.

While the arguments for common latent phenomena are well made, there remain concerns about the proposed nomenclature. As with the diagnosis of anxious depression, the presence of differing criteria between ICD-11 and ICD-11 PHC may be confusing to primary care practitioners and adversely affect opportunities for integration between primary care and specialist services. Moreover, what BSS's, BDD's, and DSM-5's somatic symptom disorder all have in common is that they confer diagnostic certainty on a set of problems that are characterized by uncertainty. They also place the locus of responsibility for the problem with the patient. Many primary care colleagues internationally prefer to retain the term 'medically unexplained symptoms' for two reasons: because it is a working hypothesis and is not diagnostically prescriptive; and because it locates the problem – and hence the responsibility for its resolution or mitigation – as one to be shared between patient and practitioner.[15]

Prospects

Although SNOMED CT is currently dominant (at least in the UK) as a clinical vocabulary, its lack of underlying diagnostic precision means it does not serve any useful purpose as a coherent classification system. Indeed, it may obstruct the emergence of such a system, if practitioners and policy makers continue with the assumption that one already exists.

There is an urgent need for convergence between ICPC-3, ICD-11, and ICD-11 PHC. These three (or perhaps two and a half) classification systems already have a great deal in common. Remaining differences, although sometimes keenly contested, are resolvable given willingness to discuss and negotiate. In the UK setting, there are opportunities for conversation between the Royal Colleges of Psychiatrists and GPs. Internationally, the World Health Organization may usefully enable further dialogue between, for example, WONCA and the World Psychiatric Association. The result should be both a more effective nosology and a greater integration of care between primary and specialist mental health services.

References

1. WONCA Working Party for Mental Health. (2018). Core Competencies of Family Doctors in Primary Mental Health Care. World Organization of Family Doctors. www.globalfamilydoctor.com/site/DefaultSite/filesystem/documents/Groups/Mental%20Health/Core%20competencies%20January%202018.pdf (accessed 9 September 2021).
2. NHS Digital. SNOMED-CT. https://digital.nhs.uk/services/terminology-and-classifications/snomed-ct (accessed 9 September 2021)
3. Schulz, S., Cornet, R. (2009). SNOMED CT's ontological commitment. *Nat Prec.* https://doi.org/10.1038/npre.2009.3465.1
4. Dowrick, C., Frances, A. (2013). Medicalising unhappiness: new classification of depression risks more patients being put on drug treatment from which they will not benefit. *BMJ,* **347,** f7140.
5. American Psychiatric Association. (2013). DSM-5 Criteria for Somatic Symptom Disorder 300.82 (F45.1). In *Diagnostic and Statistical Manual of Mental Disorders,* 5th ed. Arlington, VA: American Psychiatric Association.
6. International Classification for Primary Care. ICPC-3 Basic Concepts. www.icpc-3.info/ (accessed 10 September 2021)
7. Andrews, G., Kemp, A., Sunderland, M., et al. (2009). Normative data for the 12 item WHO Disability Assessment Schedule 2.0. *PLoS One,* **4,** e8343.
8. Horton, R. (2020). COVID-19 is not a pandemic. *Lancet,* **396,** 874.
9. Ziebold, C., Mari, J.J., Goldberg, D.P., et al. (2019). Diagnostic consequences of a new category of anxious depression and a reduced duration requirement for anxiety symptoms in the ICD-11 PHC. *J Affect Disord,* **245,** 120–125

10. Tyrer, P., Tyrer, H., Johnson, T., Yang, M. (2022). Thirty-year outcome of anxiety and depressive disorders and personality status: comprehensive evaluation of mixed symptoms and the general neurotic syndrome in the follow-up of a randomised controlled trial. *Psychol Med*, **52**, 3999–4008.

11. Goldberg, D.P., Lam, T.P., Minhas, F., et al. (2017). Primary care physicians' use of the proposed classification of common mental disorders for ICD-11. *Fam Pract*, **34**, 574–580.

12. Goldberg, D.P., Reed, G.M., Robles, R., et al. (2016). Multiple somatic symptoms in primary care: a field study for ICD-11 PHC, WHO's revised classification of mental disorders in primary care settings. *J Psychosom Res*, **91**, 48–54.

13. Ziebold, C., Goldberg, D.P., Reed, G.M., et al. (2019). Dimensional analysis of depressive, anxious and somatic symptoms presented by primary care patients and their relationship with ICD-11 PHC proposed diagnoses. *Psychol Med*, **49**, 764–771.

14. Katerndahl, D.A., Larme, A.C., Palmer, R.F., Amodei, N. (2005). Reflections on DSM classification and its utility in primary care: case studies in 'mental disorders'. *Prim Care Companion J Clin Psychiatry*, **7**, 91–99.

15. Olde Hartman, T., Lam, C.L., Usta, J., et al. (2018). Addressing the needs of patients with medically unexplained symptoms: 10 key messages. *Br J Gen Pract*, **68**, 442–443.

Index

ACE model
  depressive episode, 40, 44, 45, 49, 52
  manic episode, 43, 45
  mixed mood states, 52
acute and transient psychotic disorder (ATPD), 27–28, 30–31
  DSM-5 vs. ICD-11, 34
  vs. schizophrenia, 32
ADHD. *See* attention deficit hyperactivity disorder
adjustment disorder (AjD), 64, 67
  relation to ICD-10 and DSM-5, 65
  relation to normality and other disorders, 64
  response to criticism of Allen Frances, 65
advantages of ICD-11 classification, 35–36, 94–96
comorbidities recognition, 95
impairment of function, 94
lifespan strategy, 94, 96
qualifiers, 94–95
agoraphobia, 100
AjD. *See* adjustment disorder
Alternative Model for Personality Disorders (AMPD), 114
Anxiety and Fear-Related Disorders, 97–101, 106–107
  agoraphobia, 100
  generalized anxiety disorder (GAD), 99–100
  meta-structure, 97–98
  panic disorder, 100
  selective mutism, 101
  separation anxiety disorder, 101
  social anxiety disorder, 101
  specific phobia, 101

anxious depression, primary care mental health classifications, 141
ATPD. *See* acute and transient psychotic disorder
attention deficit hyperactivitydisorder (ADHD), 89
  DSM-5 vs. ICD-11, 93
  vs. bipolar disorder, 44
  vs. depressive episode, 42
  vs. manic episode, 45
autism spectrum disorders, 88–89
  DSM-5 vs. ICD-11, 93
  intellectual development disorders, 125–126

BDD. *See* body dysmorphic disorder
BED. *See* Binge Eating Disorder
behavioral addictions, 19–20
  substance use diagnosis, 83
Binge Eating Disorder (BED), 8, 22, 140
bipolar 'hoo' disorder, 57–58
bipolar disorder, vs. attention deficit hyperactive disorder, 44
bipolar II disorder, 21, 50–51, 57–58
bodily stress syndrome (BSS), primary care mental health classifications, 141–143
body dysmorphic disorder (BDD), 102–103
Body Integrity Dysphoria, 20
body-focused repetitive behaviour disorders, 106
borderline personality disorder, 116
BSS. *See* bodily stress syndrome

CAMHS. *See* Child and Adolescent Mental Health Services
catatonia, 22
catatonic states, 88
CDDR. *See* Clinical Descriptions and Diagnostic Requirements
CdLS. *See* Cornelia de Lange syndrome
Child and Adolescent Mental Health Services (CAMHS), 95
classification
  advantages of ICD-11 classification, 35–36, 94–96
  classificatory system tensions, 49
  schizophrenia or other primary psychotic disorders, 26–28
Clinical Descriptions and Diagnostic Requirements (CDDR)
  development of the ICD-11, 5–7
  goal of the ICD-11 CDDG development process, 36
Mental, Behavioural, and Neurodevelopmental Disorders (MBND), 7–8
co-morbidities recognition, advantage of ICD-11 classification, 95
co-morbidities, schizophrenia or other primary psychotic disorders, 32–33
comparison with DSM-5 equivalent diagnoses, 92–94
Complex PTSD (CPTSD), 10, 19, 60–62, 66–67 *See also* post-traumatic stress disorder
essential and associated features, 60–61

145

Index

Complex PTSD (cont.)
  relation to ICD-10 and DSM-5, 62
  relation to normality and other disorders, 61–62
  response to criticism of Allen Frances, 61
  terminology, 19
compulsive sexual behaviour disorder, 11, 20
conduct-dissocial disorder, 90–91
  differential diagnosis, 91
  qualifiers, 90
Cornelia de Lange syndrome (CdLS), 88
CPTSD. See Complex PTSD
cyclothymic disorder, 48

delusional disorder, 28, 31
  vs. schizophrenia, 32
delusions, manic episode, 44
depressive episode, 40–43
  ACE model, 40, 44, 45, 49, 52
  bereavement vs. depression, 42–43
  cognitive-behavioural cluster, 40–41
  developmental aspects, 42
  emptiness, sense of, 41
  features, 40–42
  grief vs. depression, 42–43
  irritability, 41
  neurovegetative cluster, 40–41
  severity and psychotic symptoms specifiers, 42
  threshold, 42–43
  vs. attention deficit hyperactivity disorder, 42
development of the ICD-11, 5–7
  Clinical Descriptions and Diagnostic Requirements (CDDR), 5–7
  context, 5
  Mental, Behavioural, and Neurodevelopmental Disorders (MBND), 5–7
  WHO implementation of ICD-11, 5
developmental language disorder, 87, 126
  DSM-5 vs. ICD-11, 92–93

developmental learning disorder, 87, 126
developmental motor co-ordination disorder, 88
developmental speech and language disorders, 92–93, 126
developmental speech fluency disorder, 87
developmental speech sound disorders, 87
Diagnostic and Statistical Manual of Mental Disorders, Fifth Edition (DSM-5)
  DSM-5 equivalent diagnoses of schizophrenia, 33–34
  DSM-5 vs. ICD-11, 17–24, 33–34, 92–94
  DSM-5 vs. ICD-11, acute and transient psychotic disorder, 34
  DSM-5 vs. ICD-11, attention deficit hyperactivity disorder, 93
  DSM-5 vs. ICD-11, autism spectrum disorders, 93
  DSM-5 vs. ICD-11, developmental language disorder, 92–93
  DSM-5 vs. ICD-11, disruptive/dissocial disorders, 93–94
  post-traumatic stress disorder, (PTSD), 7
  primary care mental health classifications, 138–139
differential diagnosis
  conduct-dissocial disorder, 91
  intellectual development disorders, 125–126
  manic episode, 45
  oppositional defiant disorder, 90
  schizophrenia or other primary psychotic disorders, 31–32
dimensional approaches, Mental, Behavioural, and Neurodevelopmental Disorders (MBND), 12
disinhibited social engagement disorder, 65

Disorders Specifically Associated with Stress, 59–67
disruptive mood dysregulation disorder (DMDD), 54
disruptive/dissocial disorders, 89–98
  changes from close or equivalent ICD-10 disorders, 91
  DSM-5 vs. ICD-11, 93–94
  redistribution of specific ICD10 childhood categories, 91
distractibility, manic episode, 44
DMDD. See disruptive mood dysregulation disorder
DSM-5. See *Diagnostic and Statistical Manual of Mental Disorders*, Fifth Edition
dysthymic disorder, 47

eating disorders
  binge eating disorder (BED), 8, 22, 140
  primary care mental health classifications, 140–141
  response to Professor Frances, 135
emptiness, sense of in a depressive episode, 41
epilepsy, 88
Episode of Harmful Substance Use (diagnosis), 75–76
excoriation disorder, 106

field testing of ICD-11 MBND, 7–8, 36
Global Clinical Practice Network (GCPN), 7
Fragile X syndrome (FXS), 88

GAD. See generalized anxiety disorder
gaming disorder, 10–11, 20, 83
GCPN. See Global Clinical Practice Network
gender identity, Mental, Behavioural, and Neurodevelopmental Disorders (MBND), 13
generalized anxiety disorder (GAD), 99–100

Global Clinical Practice
    Network (GCPN), field
    testing of ICD-11
    MBND, 7

hallucinations, manic
    episode, 44
Harmful Pattern of Substance
    Use (diagnosis), 75
Harmful Substance Use
    (diagnosis), 75
Hazardous Substance Use
    (diagnosis), 74
health anxiety disorder
    (hypochondriasis),
    104–105
hoarding disorder, 23, 105
hypochondriasis (health
    anxiety disorder), 104–105
hypomanic episode, 45–46
    developmental
        considerations, 46
    diagnostic boundaries, 46
    vs. manic episode, 45

ICPC-3. *See* International
    Classification for Primary
    Care
impairment of function,
    advantage of ICD-11
    classification, 94
intellectual development
    disorders, 122–133
    advantages of ICD-11,
        128–129
    aetiologies, 124
    autism spectrum disorder,
        125–126
    changes from ICD-10,
        126–127
    co-morbidities, 124–125
    comparison with DSM-5,
        127–128
    developmental learning
        disorder, 126
    developmental speech and
        language disorders, 126
    diagnostic boundaries from
        normality and other
        disorders, 125–126
    differential diagnosis,
        125–126
    essential features, 122–124
    other mental, behavioural, or
        neurodevelopmental
        disorders, 126, 132

physical disorders, 124
problem behaviours,
    129–132
International Classification for
    Primary Care (ICPC-3),
    139–140
International Classification of
    Diseases for Primary Care
    (ICD-11 PHC)
    convergence between
        ICPC-3, ICD-11 and
        ICD-11 PHC, 143
    reason for encounter (RFE),
        139, 140
irritability
    depressive episode, 41
    manic episode, 44

language disorders
    developmental language
        disorder, 87, 126
    developmental language
        disorder, DSM-5 vs.
        ICD-11, 92–93
    developmental speech and
        language disorders,
        92–93, 126
    developmental speech
        fluency disorder, 87
    developmental speech sound
        disorders, 87
    intellectual development
        disorders, developmental
        speech and language
        disorders, 126
    neurodevelopmental
        disorders, speech or
        language disorders, 87
    secondary speech or
        language syndrome, 87
    speech or language
        disorders, 87
lifespan strategy, advantage of
    ICD-11 classification,
    94, 96
longitudinal perspective, mood
    disorders, 55

manic episode, 43–47
    ACE model, 43, 45
    boundaries, diagnostic, 45
    delusions, 44
    developmental aspects, 44
    diagnostic boundaries, 45
    differential diagnosis, 45
    distractibility, 44

features, 43–44
hallucinations, 44
irritability, 44
vs. attention deficit
    hyperactivity disorder, 45
vs. hypomanic episode, 45
vs. mixed episode, 45, 46–47
mental health classifications,
    primary care. *See* primary
    care, mental health
    classifications
Mental, Behavioural, and
    Neurodevelopmental
    Disorders (MBND), 5–15
    advantages of ICD-11
        classification, 35–36
    Clinical Descriptions and
        Diagnostic Requirements
        (CDDR), 7–8
    Complex PTSD, 10
    compulsive sexual behaviour
        disorder, 11, 20
    development of the ICD-
        11, 5–7
    dimensional approaches, 12
    field testing of ICD-11
        MBND, 7–8
    gaming disorder, 10–11,
        20, 83
    gender identity, 13
    innovations, 12–13
    mind–body split, 12
    new disorder categories/
        diagnoses, 8–15
    next steps, 13
    prolonged grief disorder, 10
    removed disorder
        categories, 11
    substance use, 12
mind–body split, Mental,
    Behavioural, and
    Neurodevelopmental
    Disorders (MBND), 12
mixed episode, 46–47
    vs. manic episode, 45, 46–47
mixed mood states, 51–52
    ACE model, 52
MMS. *See* Mortality and
    Morbidity Statistics
mood disorders, 54–55 *See also*
    specific mood disorders
    definitions, 39
    in youth, 53–54
    longitudinal perspective, 55
    RANZCP guidelines, 49, 51
    structure of ICD-11, 39

Index

mood disorders (cont.)
  symptoms, 49–50
  terminology, 39
Mortality and Morbidity Statistics (MMS) of ICD-11, schizophrenia or other primary psychotic disorders, 27–37

neurodevelopmental disorders, 86–89, 91–96
  developmental learning disorder, 87
  developmental motor co-ordination disorder, 88
  primary tics or tic disorders, 88
  speech or language disorders, 87
  stereotyped movement disorder, 88
new disorder categories/diagnoses, 17–18
Mental, Behavioural, and Neurodevelopmental Disorders (MBND), 8–15

Obsessive-Compulsive and Related Disorders (OCRDs), 97–98, 102–107
  body dysmorphic disorder (BDD), 102–103
  body-focused repetitive behaviour disorders, 106
  conceptual approach, 106–107
  hoarding disorder, 105
  hypochondriasis (health anxiety disorder), 104–105
  meta-structure, 97–98
  obsessive-compulsive disorder (OCD), 97–98, 102
  olfactory reference disorder (ORD), 102, 103–104
  response to Allen Frances, 106
  Tourette syndrome, 105–106
obsessive-compulsive disorder (OCD), 97–98, 102
OCD. See obsessive-compulsive disorder
OCRDs. See Obsessive-Compulsive and Related Disorders

olfactory reference disorder (ORD), 102, 103–104
oppositional defiant disorder, 90
  differential diagnosis, 90
  qualifiers, 90
ORD. See olfactory reference disorder

panic disorder, 100
persistent depressive disorder (PDD), 48
personality disorder, 20–21, 52–53, 110–128
  Alternative Model for Personality Disorders (AMPD), 114
  Anankastia Domain Qualifier, 114–116
  borderline personality disorder, 116
  complexity, 110
  dimensional distribution, 110
  empirical foundation of trait domain qualifiers, 113
  future diagnosis, 117–120
  ICD-11 classification system, 111
  implications for treatment: clinical utility, 116–117
  Oltmanns & Widiger: PiCD, 114
  personality difficulty vs. personality disorder, 111–112
  Personality Inventory for DSM-5, Brief Form Plus (PID5BF+), 114
  Personality Inventory for ICD-11 (PiCD), 114
  personality trait domain qualifiers, 112–113
  personality trait domains, measuring, 113–122
  severity, 111
  severity vs. type, 110
Personality Inventory for DSM-5, Brief Form Plus (PID5BF+), 114
Personality Inventory for ICD-11 (PiCD), 114
PGD. See prolonged grief disorder
PiCD. See Personality Inventory for ICD-11

PID5BF+. See Personality Inventory for DSM-5, Brief Form Plus
post-traumatic stress disorder (PTSD), 6–7, 59–60, 66–67
  See also Complex PTSD
  co-morbidity, 60
  core elements, 59
  Diagnostic and Statistical Manual of Mental Disorders, Fifth Edition (DSM-5), 7
  relation to ICD-10 and DSM-5, 60
  relation to normality and other disorders, 60
  symptoms, 59
Premenstrual Dysphoric Disorder, 22
primary care, mental health classifications, 137–143
  anxious depression, 141
  bodily stress syndrome (BSS), 141–143
  convergence between ICPC-3, ICD-11 and ICD-11 PHC, 143
  Diagnostic and Statistical Manual of Mental Disorders, Fifth Edition (DSM-5), 138–139
  eating disorders, 140–141
  ICD-11 PHC, 140
  International Classification for Primary Care (ICPC-3), 139–140
  need for mental health classification in primary care, 137
  Systematized Nomenclature of Medicine Clinical Terms (SNOMED CT), 138, 143
  World Organization of Family Doctors (WONCA), 137
primary tics or tic disorders, 88
prolonged grief disorder (PGD), 10, 18, 62–64, 67
  essential and associated features, 62–63
  relation to ICD-10 and DSM-5, 64
  relation to normality and other disorders, 63

response to criticism of Allen Frances, 63
PTSD. *See* post-traumatic stress disorder

qualifiers
  advantage of ICD-11 classification, 94–95
  conduct-dissocial disorder, 90
  oppositional defiant disorder, 90
  substance use, 81–82

RAD. *See* reactive attachment disorder
RANZCP mood disorders guidelines, 49, 51
reactive attachment disorder (RAD), 65–66
reason for encounter (RFE), International Classification for Primary Care, 139, 140

schizoaffective disorder, 27, 30, 34
  vs. schizophrenia, 31
schizophrenia or other primary psychotic disorders, 25–38
  acute and transient psychotic disorder (ATPD), 27–28, 30–31, 34
  acute and transient psychotic disorder (ATPD) vs, schizophrenia, 32
  Bleuler, Eugen, 25–26
  boundaries, diagnostic, 31
  characteristics, 26, 28
  classical schizophrenia subtypes, 27
  classification, 26–28
  co-morbidities, 32–33
  course of schizophrenia, 30
  delusional disorder, 28, 31
  delusional disorder vs. schizophrenia, 32
  diagnosis, 29
  diagnostic boundaries, 31
  differential diagnosis, 31–32
  DSM-5 equivalent diagnoses, 33–34
  essential features, 28–31
  Kraepelin, Emil, 25

Mortality and Morbidity Statistics (MMS) of ICD-11, 27–37
  onset age, 30
  origins of the concept of schizophrenia, 25–26
  overall structure for the ICD-11 section, 27–37
  schizoaffective disorder, 27, 30, 34
  schizoaffective disorder vs schizophrenia, 31
  schizotypal disorder, 28, 30
  schizotypal disorder vs. schizophrenia, 32
  Schneider, Kurt, 26
  structural changes of psychotic disorders from ICD-10 to ICD-11, 28
  symptoms, 29–30
  terminology, 25
schizophreniform disorder, 34
schizotypal disorder, 28, 30
  vs. schizophrenia, 32
secondary speech or language syndrome, 87
selective mutism, 101
separation anxiety disorder, 101
SNOMED CT. *See* Systematized Nomenclature of Medicine Clinical Terms
social anxiety disorder, 101
social disorders. *See* conduct-dissocial disorder, disinhibited social engagement disorder, disruptive/dissocial disorders
specific phobia, 101
speech or language disorders. *See* language disorders
stereotyped movement disorder, 88
stress. *See also* adjustment disorder, Complex PTSD, disinhibited social engagement disorder, post-traumatic stress disorder, prolonged grief

disorder, reactive attachment disorder
Disorders Specifically Associated with Stress, 59–67
  measurement tools, 67
  questionnaires, 67
Substance Dependence (diagnosis), 76–78
  additional substance use diagnoses in ICD-11, 78–79
  comparisons with ICD-10 and DSM-5, 78
  components, 76–77
  conceptual definition, 76
  key features, 76
Substance Dependence and Harm, 77
Substance Intoxication, 79
Substance Withdrawal, 79
substance use, 70–84
  aims of this chapter, 70–71
  background and input to ICD-11, 71–72
  behavioral addictions, 83
  brain processes, 82
  cultural specificity, 82
  diagnosis, 72–83
  disorders due to use of other substances, 81
  Episode of Harmful Substance Use (diagnosis), 75–76
  gap between the two major classification systems, 83
  Harmful Pattern of Substance Use (diagnosis), 75
  Harmful Substance Use (diagnosis), 75
  Hazardous Substance Use (diagnosis), 74
  hierarchy of substance use and disorder, 73–74
  level of alcohol use, 82
  Mental, Behavioural, and Neurodevelopmental Disorders (MBND), 12
  nonspecific consequences, 82
  primary diagnoses, 74–76
  range of substances, 72–74
  reactions to the ICD-11 substance diagnoses and comments from Allen Frances, 82–83

substance use (cont.)
  selected statistics, 70
  Substance Dependence (diagnosis), 76–78
  substance-induced mental disorders, 79–80
  substance-induced neurocognitive disorders, 80–81
  subtypes and qualifiers within ICD-11, 81–82
  use of ICD-11 in primarry care, 83
  World Health Organization (WHO), public health approach, 70
Systematized Nomenclature of Medicine Clinical Terms (SNOMED CT), 138

terminology
  mood disorders, 39
  schizophrenia or other primary psychotic disorders, 25
tics
  primary tics or tic disorders, 88
Tourette syndrome, 105–106
trichotillomania, 106
tuberous sclerosis, 88

WHO. *See* World Health Organization
WONCA. *See* World Organization of Family Doctors
World Health Organization (WHO)
  implementation of ICD-11, 5
  substance use, public health approach, 70
World Organization of Family Doctors (WONCA)
  primary care mental health classifications, 137